Neuropsychiatric Dementias

CLINICAL INSIGHTS

Neuropsychiatric Dementias

Edited by
DILIP V. JESTE, M.D.

Chief, Unit on Movement Disorders and Dementia, Neuropsychiatry Branch, National Institute of Mental Health, Saint Elizabeths Hospital, Washington, D.C.

AMERICAN PSYCHIATRIC PRESS, INC.
Washington, D.C.

Note: The authors have worked to ensure that all information in this book concerning drug dosages, schedules, and routes of administration is accurate at the time of publication and consistent with standards set by the U.S. Food and Drug Administration and the general medical community. As medical research and practice advance, however, therapeutic standards may change. For this reason and because human and mechanical errors sometimes occur, we recommend that readers follow the advice of a physician directly involved in their care or the care of a member of their family.

Manufactured in the U.S.A.

The paper used in this publication meets the minimum requirements of American National Standard for Information Sciences—Permanence of Paper for Printed Library Materials, ANSI Z39.48-1984. ∞™

Library of Congress Cataloging in Publication Data

Main entry under title:

Neuropsychiatric dementias.

(Clinical insights)
Includes bibliographies.
1. Dementia. 2. Brain—Diseases—Age factors.
3. Neuropsychiatry. I. Jeste, Dilip V. II. Series.
[DNLM: 1. Dementia. WM 220 N493]
RC521.N48 1986 616.89'83 86-10734
ISBN 0-88048-087-4 (soft: alk. paper)

Contents

Contributors

Gerard Addonizio, M.D.
Assistant Professor of Psychiatry, New York Hospital–Cornell Medical Center, Westchester Division, White Plains, New York

D. Frank Benson, M.D.
The Augustus S. Rose Professor of Neurology, School of Medicine, University of California, Los Angeles

Karen Faith Berman, M.D.
Staff Psychiatrist, Neuropsychiatry Branch, National Institute of Mental Health, Saint Elizabeths Hospital, Washington, D.C.

Jean Lud Cadet, M.D.
Staff Psychiatrist, Neuropsychiatry Branch, National Institute of Mental Health, Saint Elizabeths Hospital, Washington, D.C.

Jeffrey L. Cummings, M.D.
Assistant Professor, Department of Neurology, School of Medicine, University of California, Los Angeles

Dilip V. Jeste, M.D.
Chief, Unit on Movement Disorders and Dementia, Neuropsychiatry Branch, National Institute of Mental Health, Saint Elizabeths Hospital, Washington, D.C.

James B. Lohr, M.D.
Staff Psychiatrist, Neuropsychiatry Branch, National Institute of Mental Health, Saint Elizabeths Hospital, Washington, D.C.

Carol Ludwig, M.D.
Assistant Professor, Department of Neurology, George Washington University Medical Center, Washington, D.C.

Ranjit B. Mani, M.D.
Clinical and Research Fellow, Department of Neurology, Massachusetts General Hospital, Boston

Carol A. Overman, Ph.D.
Speech Pathologist, Department of Speech Pathology and Audiology, Saint Elizabeths Hospital, Washington, D.C.

Charles A. Shamoian, M.D.
Professor of Psychiatry, New York Hospital–Cornell Medical Center, Westchester Division, White Plains, New York

David Shore, M.D.
Chief, Biological and Clinical Factors Research Program, Division of Clinical Research, National Institute of Mental Health, Rockville, Maryland

Mark Tecco
Surgical Transplant Division, Department of Surgery, George Washington University Hospital, Washington, D.C.

Daniel R. Weinberger, M.D.
Chief, Section on Clinical Neuropsychiatry, Neuropsychiatry Branch, National Institute of Mental Health, Saint Elizabeths Hospital, Washington, D.C.

Richard Jed Wyatt, M.D.
Chief, Neuropsychiatry Branch, National Institute of Mental Health, Saint Elizabeths Hospital, Washington, D.C.

Introduction

With the graying of America, dementia has assumed epidemic proportions. When we add dementias associated with certain psychiatric disorders to the dementias of the elderly, the severity of the overall problem becomes even more apparent. Fortunately, advances in related basic and clinical sciences are helping us know more about the various dementing disorders than ever before. Although we still have a long way to go before arriving at solutions to major dementias, we are at least marching in the right direction.

This monograph includes contributions from investigators in the fields of neurology, psychiatry, and neuropathology. Principal neurologic as well as psychiatric disorders associated with dementia are considered, although this is not meant to be an exhaustive treatise on dementia as such. In Chapter 1, Drs. Frank Benson and Jeffrey Cummings present a clinical scheme for diagnosis and differential diagnosis of various dementias. The emphasis is on detecting the small but significant minority of reversible dementias. In Chapter 2, Dr. David Shore, Dr. Carol Overman, Mark Tecco, and Dr. Richard Wyatt describe the features of the most

---

Dr. Jeste is now the director of the neuropsychiatry program and neuropathology research laboratory at the University of California at San Diego.

common dementia—Alzheimer's disease—and discuss their own longitudinal follow-up study of patients with this disorder. The recommendations for using specific tests and retests to separate dementias that do not worsen with time are of clinical value. In Chapter 3, Drs. Karen Berman and Daniel Weinberger review the conceptual background of schizophrenic dementia. Their studies of regional cerebral blood flow, suggesting an association between prefrontal pathology and the "dementia praecox," are of interest. Drs. Gerard Addonizio and Charles Shamoian present in Chapter 4 an overview of the vast but often confusing literature on the relationship between depression and dementia. They then offer clinical recommendations for workup of patients whose affective and cognitive symptoms pose diagnostic dilemmas. Finally, in Chapter 5, Drs. James Lohr, Ranjit Mani, Jean Cadet, and Carol Ludwig and I discuss studies of neuronal loss in specific areas of the brain in normal aging and in certain dementias. The relatively selective vulnerabilities of catecholamine-rich regions to aging-related neuronal drop-out and of cholinergic neurons in the basal forebrain to certain dementing disorders deserve further research.

Dilip V. Jeste, M.D.

1

A Scheme to Differentiate the Dementias

D. Frank Benson, M.D.
Jeffrey L. Cummings, M.D.

1

A Scheme to Differentiate the Dementias

With the "graying of America," the rapidly increasing number of elderly, the incidence of dementia is also on the rise. It is estimated that significant disabling dementia occurs in 5 to 20 percent of individuals over 65 years of age (Broe et al. 1976; Kaye et al. 1970), depending primarily on definition. In terms of the total health care dollars needed for its care, dementia now ranks among the leaders, cancer and cardiovascular disease. Cost is not the only factor; the misery and social problems of demented individuals and their families as well as the demands on community resources warrant attention. Dementia has truly become a major public health problem of contemporary society (Katzman and Karasu 1975).

One recognized cause of dementia is Alzheimer's disease, which is now considered the single most frequent cause of dementia in the elderly (Katzman 1976; Plum 1979). This concept was strengthened by the work of Roth et al. (1966), who noted that the neuropathologic alterations characteristic of Alzheimer's disease (senile plaques, neurofibrillary tangles, and granuovacuolar degeneration) showed a quantitative correlation with the severity of dementia in a series of carefully studied elderly individuals. Many clinicians now accept that most dementia in the elderly is dementia of the Alzheimer type (DAT). Most studies recognize, however, that a great percentage of demented individuals over 65 years of age suffer from disorders other than DAT, although many of these disorders meet the nonspecific criteria used for DAT diagnosis. Follow-up studies of patients diagnosed as suffering from DAT have shown error rates of 18 to 57 percent (Kendell 1974; Nott and Fleminger 1975; Ron et al. 1979; Sulkava et al. 1983). This overdiagnosis of DAT may have tragic consequences because many non-DAT dementias are completely or partially treatable (Benson 1982; Wells 1977), and misidentification as DAT may prematurely terminate the search for potentially reversible causes of the intellectual deterioration.

One basic reason for poor recognition of causes of dementia stems from the long-standing belief that Alzheimer's disease is a neuropathologic diagnosis, a disorder that can be suspected by the clinician but diagnosed only postmortem. Most definitions of DAT are notably nonspecific and tend to emphasize the exclusion of other disorders (see the *Diagnostic and Statistical Manual of Mental Disorders [Third Edition]*, American Psychiatric Association 1980). A need for positive clinical criteria for the diagnosis of Alzheimer's disease is recognized (McKhann et al. 1984). A simplified scheme to approach this problem is now presented.

DIAGNOSTIC SCHEME

Figure 1 depicts a flow sheet that can be used by the clinician when evaluating a patient with dementia. Each step outlined in this diagram uses clinical information, reserving the laboratory techniques for confirmation. The steps in the scheme are overlapping, however, and need not be carried out formally or in the exact order presented in Figure 1. If each of the major categories is kept in mind and appropriate studies performed to rule in or rule out these types of dementia, the clinician will have a far better chance of discovering cases of treatable dementia.

Step 1 is to demonstrate that dementia may be present and that a full-scale dementia evaluation is indicated. This state can be determined by fulfilling clinical criteria, the results of an abbreviated mental status evaluation or both.

The next step is to seek the presence of one of the cortical dementing disorders (Alzheimer's or Pick's disease). This step can be performed with fairly consistent accuracy by using the profile of features for the diagnosis of DAT presented in Table 1 later in this chapter. In the very early and the late stages of these disorders, the guidelines presented by the profile are less precise, and additional clinical history and considerable experience is necessary for an accurate diagnosis. Most patients who are seen with either Alzheimer- or Pick-type dementia are in the middle stage of these

Figure 1. Diagnostic scheme for dementias.

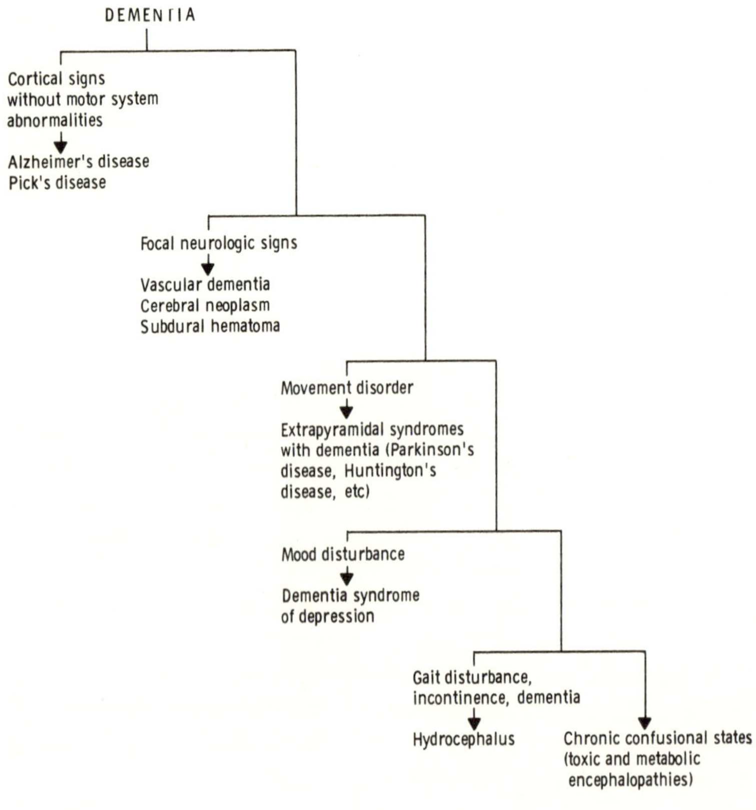

disorders, and the profile has considerable potential for providing an accurate clinical diagnosis.

If the patient has been shown to be demented but evidence does not suggest one of the cortical dementias, the next step is to rule out the presence of vascular dementia. Again, a clinical examination combined with the use of a cerebral ischemia inventory provides a relatively accurate determination (Hachinski et al. 1975). The presence of a dementing condition, the absence of findings of cortical dementia, and a high score on the cerebral ischemia inventory would strongly suggest a vascular cause for the dementia.

The next step is to rule out one of the major movement disorders frequently associated with dementia. This is best done by observation because Huntington's disease, Parkinson's disease, and Wilson's disease, among others, are best determined clinically. Formal screening tests for movement disorders are available to quantitate the abnormalities, but most are designed to seek drug-induced dyskinesias. Clinical evaluation remains the best means of detecting the movement disorders that may accompany dementia.

Step 5 is to rule out depression as a cause of dementia; this is based on clinical impression abetted, if necessary, by questionnaires. Depressive (pseudo) dementia is not common, but it represents a treatable cause of acquired cognitive disorder and deserves consideration.

Finally, having excluded all of these possibilities in a patient who is demented, the sizable number of disorders that can produce a chronic confusional state must be considered. It is impossible to present a simple scheme to diagnose the hundreds of causes of chronic confusion, but if the other types of dementia have been ruled out, the clinician's attention can be directed to these disorders. Although few of the other causes of dementia can be diagnosed with laboratory studies, a wide variety of laboratory tests may be useful in diagnosing chronic confusional states. Many of the disorders in this category respond to appropriate therapy.

Specific directions for performing each step in the dementia diagnostic flow scheme are now presented.

DETERMINATION OF DEMENTIA

To determine the presence of dementia with at least sufficient accuracy for clinical purposes, several steps can be taken. First, and most valuable, is demonstration that the patient does have an alteration in intellectual capacity. By generally accepted definition, dementia is an impairment of intellectual competency sufficient to interfere with normal living. For diagnostic purposes, we (Cummings and Benson 1983; Cummings et al. 1980) suggest that dementia be defined as sustained impairment of intellectual competency that includes significant performance disorder in at least three of the following spheres: speech and/or language, memory, cognition, visuospatial skills, or personality. This definition stresses the presence of a sustained mental disturbance; an acute intellectual impairment is better called delirium or acute confusion and will have different causes and treatments. In addition, the definition emphasizes that demonstration of acquired impairment in at least three major intellectual functions warrants a clinical suspicion of dementia. Serious disturbance in only a single area such as language (aphasia) or memory (amnesia) in the face of normal or near-normal performance in other areas should not be considered dementia.

A number of tests can confirm the clinical impression of dementia, among them the Mini-Mental State Exam (Folstein et al. 1975), the Blessed Dementia Scale (Blessed et al. 1968), and the Clinical Dementia Rating Scale (CDR) (Hughes et al. 1982). Unfortunately, no test is consistently accurate, and all must be used with caution. Most deal with only a limited number of intellectual activities (for example, language or memory), and normal scores can be achieved in the face of significant dementia. Some (for example, CDR, Blessed Scale) combine an assessment of impairment in daily living activities with a quantification of intellectual competency. Although more inclusive, these scales only roughly indicate mental impairment. A clinical impression of dementia can be supported by one or more such tests, and further efforts to identify the cause of the dementia can be initiated.

DIAGNOSIS OF CORTICAL DEGENERATIVE DEMENTIA

Degenerative diseases involving the cerebral hemispheres that produce dementia become manifest in one of two anatomic patterns. DAT and Pick-type dementia affect the cerebral cortex far more than the subcortical structures; other degenerative diseases such as Huntington's disease, Parkinson's disease, and other extrapyramidal disorders that can cause dementia (discussed later) greatly affect the function of the basal ganglia and thalamus and have relatively limited affect on the cerebral cortex (Benson 1983). Most of these degenerative diseases lack pathognomonic laboratory features, but subcortical degenerative processes produce characteristic movement disturbances (for example, chorea, rigidity, tremor, and bradykinesia) that allow clinical recognition. Cortical degenerative diseases are evidenced solely by the mental status alterations they produce.

Improvement in the accuracy of the clinical diagnosis of DAT depends on the establishment of restrictive clinical criteria sufficiently characteristic of DAT to distinguish it from other dementing disorders. We have suggested (Cummings and Benson 1983) that DAT produces a distinct profile of findings that is clinically identifiable and that differentiates DAT from non-DAT dementias. Using the operationalized definitions for each component of the profile (see Table 1), we (Cummings and Benson 1986) found a statistically significant difference between the scores of the DAT and non-DAT causes of dementia ($p < .005$). The profile includes memory disturbances, aphasia, visuospatial abnormalities, cognitive disturbances, and personality alterations progressing insidiously in a patient with normal posture, gait, coordination, psychomotor speed, and speech articulation. These characteristics were chosen from descriptions of previously reported autopsy-proven cases of DAT with clinical and neuropsychologic studies. The profile emphasizes abnormal intellectual functions and normal motor functions, a clinical pattern emphasized by Alzheimer in the first report of the disease (Alzheimer 1907/1977).

Memory is profoundly disturbed in DAT and is one of the most

Table 1. Profile of Clinical Features Differentiating DAT From Other Dementias

Function	Clinical Features		
	DAT	Intermediate	Non-DAT
Memory	Disoriented; unable to remember three words for three minutes; recall not aided by prompting	Recalls one or two of three words spontaneously; incompletely aided by prompting	Normal or mild forgetfulness that improves with clues
Visuospatial	Disorganized, unrecognizable	Flattening, omissions, distortions	Normal or mildly clumsy; minimal distortions
Cognition	Fails to interpret simple proverbs or idioms; acalculia	Fails to abstract simple proverbs and has difficulty with mathematical problems	Normal or impaired cognitive abstractions and calculations
Personality	Unaware or indifferent; irritability not uncommon	Appropriately concerned	Marked personality changes or depression
Language	Fluent aphasia with anomia; decreased comprehension, paraphasia	Anomia; mild comprehension deficits may be present	Normal
Speech	Normal	Slurred, amelodic, hypophonic	Mute, severely dysarthric
Psychomotor speed	Normal, prompt answers	Hesitant replies	Slow, long latency to response
Posture	Normal, erect	Stooped	Abnormal, flexed, or extended
Gait	Normal	Shuffling	Hemiparetic, ataxic, apractic, or hyperkinetic
Movements	Normal	Imprecise, uncoordinated	Tremor, akinesia, rigidity, or chorea

DAT = dementia of the Alzheimer type.

consistent clinical features of the disease. The learning of new information is impaired early in the course and reflects a disturbance in the ability to encode the stimulus material for later retrieval (Davis and Mumford 1984; Miller 1971, 1972; Shuttleworth 1982). Recollection of remote memories is also impaired and, by the midphase, DAT patients have little recall.

Aphasia has received less attention as a characteristic of DAT, but recent studies suggest that language disturbances are a consistent feature of the disorder (Appell et al. 1982; Bayles 1982; Cummings et al. 1985; Martin and Fedio 1983; Schwartz et al. 1979; Skelton-Robinson and Jones 1984). In the early stages of the disease, the patient has an empty verbal output (low information content) and may be unable to name some stimulus items correctly. As the disease progresses, the patient manifests a fluent aphasia with impaired comprehension and preserved repetition resembling transcortical sensory aphasia. In the final stages, the predominant verbal output is echolalia, palilalia, or mutism (Cummings and Benson 1983; Cummings et al. 1985).

Visuospatial disturbances are evident early in the course. Elementary visual perception remains unaffected, but analysis of spatial patterns and reproduction of model figures become impaired (Brouwers et al. 1984; Schlotterer et al. 1983). Standardized neuropsychologic examination reveals performance deficits on the Wechsler Adult Intelligence Scale subtests as well as on visual retention tests, the Bender Visual-Motor Gestalt Test, and trail-making tests (Berg et al. 1984; Storandt et al. 1984).

Cognitive abnormalities in DAT are manifested as difficulties in abstracting the meaning of metaphoric statements and performing arithmetic operations (Cummings and Benson 1983). In the early stages of DAT, these abnormalities are mild, but they exhibit progressive impairment as the disease advances.

Personality alterations in DAT have been more difficult to characterize, but they represent an important clinical finding. The most common change is a progressive indifference and unconcern. Despite widespread cognitive deficits and progressive deterioration, obvious to family and friends, the patient manifests little concern and is rarely anxious or seriously depressed. Of the 377

DAT patients studied by Larrsen et al. (1963), 69 percent had this "simple" type of dementia without extravagant behavioral alterations, 18 percent were paranoid, and 10 percent were depressed. A low incidence of depression among DAT patients has been confirmed by other investigators (Knesevich et al. 1983; Sulkava 1982), and when a higher prevalence has been reported the depression has been most frequent in the early stages of the disease (Reifler et al. 1982). The delusions manifested by DAT patients are usually loosely held, poorly structured persecutory beliefs involving personal danger or theft of personal goods (Cummings 1985).

In contrast to the marked intellectual deterioration, the basic sensorimotor system remains normal through most of the course of DAT. The patient's posture remains upright, the gait is spry and normal, coordination is unaffected, and psychomotor speed is unimpaired (Koller et al. 1984; Pomara et al. 1981). Myoclonus is common in later stages, but chorea, athetosis, tremor, and dystonia are rare (Faden and Townsend 1976; Jacob 1970; Mayeux et al. 1981). In the terminal phases of the disease, rigidity and flexion of the limbs is noted, and the patient eventually assumes a posture of quadriparesis in flexion.

The mechanical aspects of speech, like other motor abilities, are preserved long into the course of DAT (Cummings et al. 1985). Speech remains normal; language is progressively impaired. This contrasts with most other dementia-producing illnesses in which both speech and language are abnormal (for example, multi-infarct dementia) or speech is compromised but language is unimpaired (for example, extrapyramidal syndromes with dementia).

The characteristics discussed previously provide a distinct clinical profile that aids clinical recognition of DAT and can be correlated with the pathophysiology of DAT. Brun and Gustafson (1978) demonstrated that senile plaques and neurofibrillary tangles were most abundant in the medial temporal and the temporo-parieto-occipital junction areas. Cholinergic enzymes are also most depleted in these same regions (Davies 1978). Cerebral blood flow and cerebral cortical metabolism show a similar geographic distribution of maximum abnormalities (Benson et al. 1983; Chase et al. 1984; Foster et al. 1984; Gustafson et al. 1978). Thus, DAT affects specific regions of the brain, reflected in a distinctive, clinically identifiable clinical syndrome.

Two varieties of cortical degenerative dementias are recognized: DAT and Pick-type dementia. The latter is far less common than DAT, usually begins in late middle age, and affects women more commonly than men (Cummings and Benson 1983). Alzheimer- and Pick-type dementia share many features including age of onset, absence of sensorimotor system abnormalities, and presence of a prominent aphasia. The pattern of intellectual deficits manifested by the two disorders is distinct, however, allowing differentiation on the basis of the clinical examination (see Table 2). In contrast to the indifference manifested by DAT patients, Pick's disease patients often develop a disinhibited "frontal lobe" syndrome with poor judgment, loss of tact and concern, coarsening and facetiousness (Lishman 1978). The Klüver-Bucy syndrome (placidity, bulimia, hypersexuality, hypermetamorphosis, hyperorality, sensory agnosia) may emerge late in the course of DAT, but components of the syndrome are often prominent early in the course of Pick's disease (Cummings and Duchen 1981; Lilly et al. 1983). In DAT, memory and arithmetic and visuospatial abilities are involved early in the clinical course; in contrast, these abilities are often spared until the middle or even late stages of Pick's disease (Cummings 1982; Robertson et al. 1958; Stengel 1943;

Table 2. Clinical Features Distinguishing Dementia of the Alzheimer Type (DAT) and Pick's Disease

Clinical characteristic	DAT	Pick's disease
Personality	Indifference	Disinhibition
Klüver-Bucy syndrome	Late in course	Early in course
Language	Transcortical sensory aphasia	Stereotyped verbal output; echolalia, mutism
Memory	Abnormal early	Normal until mid or late stages
Visuospatial skills	Abnormal early	Normal until mid or late stages
Calculation	Abnormal early	Normal until mid or late stages
Computed tomographic scan	Normal or generalized atrophy	Frontotemporal atrophy

Wechsler et al. 1982). The distinguishing clinical features of Pick's disease may be supported by computed tomography (CT). Results of CT for DAT patients are normal or reveal generalized cortical atrophy, whereas in Pick's disease the CT frequently demonstrates focal frontal or temporal atrophy (Cummings and Benson 1983; Groen and Edntz 1982; McGeachie et al. 1979; Wechsler et al. 1982).

Diagnosis of Vascular Dementia

Vascular dementia (multi-infarct dementia, or MID) refers to the progressive impairment of intellectual function produced by cerebral infarction (Hachinski et al. 1974). The nature of the resulting dementia syndrome depends on the number and location of cerebral infarctions and the total volume of damaged tissue. Investigators (Hachinski et al. 1975; Rosen et al. 1980) have produced and modified clinical criteria that correlate with cerebral blood flow studies and clinical pathologic investigations indicative of MID. Table 3 summarizes these and other characteristics that we have found valuable in identifying MID. An abrupt onset and stepwise deterioration are the typical markers of recurrent cerebral infarctions. The personality may remain relatively intact, and the patient often retains insight into the progressive intellectual decline. Both depression and psychotic episodes are more common in MID than in DAT (Cummings 1985; Hachinsi et al. 1975; Tomonaga et al. 1982). Hypertension is the most common cause of MID, and multiple lacunar infarctions located in the basal ganglia, thalamus, and internal capsule are the lesions most commonly correlated with hypertensive vascular dementia. Other cardiovascular disorders including diabetes, atherosclerosis, inflammatory conditions, and embolic disorders are risk factors that increase the likelihood of vascular dementia. A history of strokes or transient ischemic attacks is common, and unilateral or bilateral neurologic signs may be evident upon examination. Computed tomography may reveal single or multiple lucencies consistent with cerebral infarctions, but the infarctions may be too small to be visualized radiologically (Ladurner at al. 1982).

The clinical findings of the dementia associated with multiple cerebral infarctions are variable, depending on the location of the hemispheric damage (Cummings and Benson 1983; Perez et al. 1975). Memory is often less impaired in MID than in DAT (Perez et al. 1976), and dysarthria is more common in MID. In most cases, the clinical features of MID are easily distinguishable from those of DAT.

Two identifiable variants of vascular dementia are Binswanger's disease and the angular gyrus syndrome. Binswanger's disease resembles other types of MID, but the infarctions are concentrated in the cerebral white matter (Caplan and Schoene 1978; De Reuck et al. 1980). Focal lucencies in the corona radiata may be demonstrated by CT (Rosenberg et al. 1979). The angular gyrus syndrome results from focal infarction in the left posterior hemisphere causing a fluent aphasia, alexia with agraphia, acalculia, right–left disorientiation, finger agnosia, and constructional disturbances (Benson et al. 1982). The multiplicity of intellectual deficits, combined with the absence of motor system abnormalities, produces a clinical syndrome that closely resembles DAT. The two can be distinguished by the awareness of language disturbance, engagement in conversation, and preservation of spatial orientiation and nonverbal memory evident in patients with angular gyrus syndrome (Benson et al. 1982).

Table 3. Clinical Features of Vascular Dementia

Abrupt onset
Stepwise deterioration
Relative preservation of personality
Depression
Psychosis
History of hypertension or other predisposing cardiovascular disease
Evidence of vascular disease outside the central nervous system
History of strokes
History of transient ischemic attacks
Focal or bilateral neurologic signs
Emotional lability (pseudobulbar palsy)
Single or multiple lucencies on computed tomographic scan (or other imaging technique)
Focal slowing on electroencephalogram

DIAGNOSIS OF EXTRAPYRAMIDAL SYNDROMES WITH DEMENTIA

Extrapyramidal syndromes that frequently accompany dementia include Huntington's disease, Parkinson's disease, progressive supranuclear palsy, Wilson's disease, spinocerebellar degeneration, thalamic degeneration, and idiopathic basal ganglia calcification (Cummings and Benson 1983). Most of these disorders can be identified clinically by characteristic movement disturbances (chorea, tremor, rigidity, bradykinesia, and ataxia) or laboratory findings (serum and urine copper abnormalities; CT evidence of caudate atrophy, lenticular nucleus lucency, or basal ganglia calcification). They represent the classic subcortical dementias (Albert et al. 1974; Cummings and Benson 1983; McHugh and Folstein 1975).

The dementia syndrome seen with the extrapyramidal disturbances differs from that of the cortical degenerative disorders (see Table 4). The subcortical disorders spare language function, cause

Table 4. Distinguishing Characteristics of Cortical and Subcortical Dementias

Characteristic	Cortical dementia	Subcortical dementia
Language	Aphasia	No aphasia
Memory	Amnesia (abnormal storage)	Forgetfulness (abnormal retrieval)
Abstraction	Impaired	Dilapidated
Calculation	Impaired	Dilapidated
Processing speed	Normal	Slowed
Personality	Indifferent or disinhibited	Apathetic
Depression	Uncommon	Common
Psychosis	Uncommon	Common
Motor system	Normal until late in course	Abnormal (for example, bradykinesia, tremor, rigidity, chorea, ataxia)
Dysarthria	Absent	Present
Causes	Alzheimer's or Pick's disease	Huntington's disease, Parkinson's disease, Wilson's disease, progressive supranuclear palsy, thalamic degeneration, spinocerebellar degeneration, basal ganglia calcification

a memory disturbance featuring poor recall rather than poor information storage, and show a less severe dilapidation of calculation and abstraction skills (Albert et al. 1974; Benson 1983; Cummings and Benson 1984; McHugh and Folstein 1975; Pearlson et al. 1981; Veroff et al. 1982). Psychomotor speed is slowed, thereby causing a prolonged central processing time and long latencies between responses, contrasting with the preserved psychomotor speed of patients with cortical degenerative diseases. Personality and neuropsychiatric disturbances are also different. The cortical diseases produce indifference or disinhibition, whereas subcortical processes feature apathy, depression, and psychosis (Albert et al. 1974; Cummings 1985; Cummings and Benson 1983, 1984; Dewhurst et al. 1969; Mayeux et al. 1981). Motor system abnormalities including dysarthria are prominent in subcortical disorders and usually occur in the late stages of cortical degeneration.

DIAGNOSIS OF DEPRESSIVE DEMENTIA

It has long been recognized that dementia occurs in some cases of severe depression (Kiloh 1961). In fact, the degree of dementia produced may be severe enough to mask the depression. Depressive dementia was originally termed depressive pseudodementia (Kiloh 1961; Post 1975), but recent interpretations suggest that this represents a true dementing condition and, as such, deserves the term dementia of depression or depressive dementia (McHugh and Folstein 1979). Although the condition clearly exists, it is not common even though depression and dementia are the most common psychiatric disorders of old age (Spar 1982). The combination, however, particularly with depression as the source of dementia, is relatively unusual. A dementia state, based on depression, does exist, and appropriate treatment often produces a remarkable reversal of the dementing picture. The diagnosis is important (see Chapter 4).

A number of key findings can lead one to suspect depressive dementia (Caine 1981; Cummings and Benson 1983; Wells 1979). Included are a relatively recent onset and rapid progression of the dementia, a past history or family history of significant affective disorder, and significant dysphoria preceding the dementing state. In most instances, psychomotor retardation is so severe that a negative, mute, nonresponding state prevails. Forgetfulness is severe, cognitive functions are seriously hindered, and the patient's verbal output is limited or absent. When a verbal response is given, the sentence rapidly dwindles in volume and often terminates before completion. Voice is soft, to the point of being incomprehensible, and the degree of hypophonia increases as the patient speaks. Depressive dementia is a clinical diagnosis, and confirmation may prove difficult (Wells 1982). Although a number of questionnaires (for example, Beck 1963; Zung 1965) and rating scales (for example, Hamilton 1967) are available and a laboratory study (Dexamethasone Suppression) may provide supportive evidence, none has proved sufficiently reliable for diagnosis. The patient may be unable or unwilling to cooperate with formal interview or questionnaire-type tests, and many nondepressed dementia patients fail to suppress cortisol. The importance of the diagnosis is apparent, however; depression often responds to current pharmaceutical therapy, and, particularly in this age group, electroshock therapy is often effective. The alteration from a helpless, seriously demented patient to a basically normal elderly individual is extremely gratifying.

DIAGNOSIS OF CHRONIC CONFUSIONAL STATE

Having failed to fulfill any of the categories described here, the patient may well have a cause of dementia outside the major categories. A catch-all term, "chronic confusional state," has been suggested. This is not a diagnostic entity; rather, it represents a collection of diverse disorders, all of which can impair mental functioning (Benson 1982). Table 5 outlines some of the many recognized causes of chronic confusional state. Although many are rare, the total group is large enough to make up a significant portion of the elderly demented population.

As could be expected from such a diverse group of clinical entities, a striking variety of clinical courses are present. Most show a slow progressive deterioration with apathy, psychomotor retardation, forgetfulness, dilapidation of cognitive function, and a relative retention of cortical functions such as language and the ability to learn new material. The diagnosis is often obvious because the disease state underlying the mental impairment is known (for example, chronic obstructive pulmonary disease and repeated bouts of cardiac arrythmia). In many instances, however, the cause is obscure, and considerable investigation is needed to discover it.

The clinical laboratory often is of far greater help in diagnosing the chronic confusional state than other causes of dementia. Both the roentgenographic CT and the electroencephalogram can present either a specific diagnosis or findings that lead to a diagnosis. Neuropsychologic testing may help by outlining specific areas of impairment. The clinical laboratory may provide considerable assistance. Appropriate tests (for example, vitamin B_{12} determination, thyroid levels, tests of heavy metals, or chemical intoxicants, may lead to a specific treatment that can produce a remarkable alteration of the dementing state. A number of the causes of chronic confusional state are treatable disorders that can be reversed or actually cured. The percentage of cases of dementia

Table 5. Chronic Confusional States (Partial Listing)

Disorder	Etiology
Systemic disorders	Pulmonary insufficiency, cardiac insufficiency, anemia, uremia, porphyria
Endocrine disorders	Panhypopituitarism, Addison's disease, myxedema, recurrent hypoglycemia
Collagen-vascular disorders	Systemic lupus erythematosus, temporal arteritis, sarcoidosis
Infectious disorders	Central nervous system syphilis, cerebral abscess, Whipple's disease, Jakob-Creutzfeldt disease, central nervous system tuberculosis
Chemical poisonings	Alcohol, organophosphates, heavy metals (arsenic, mercury, lead), trichlorethylene
Drug poisonings	Haloperidol, bromides, phenytoin, lithium, barbiturates, atropine, and related compounds
Deficiency states	Pellagra, vitamin B_{12} deficiency, folate deficiency
Intracranial masses	Meningioma, glioma, chronic subdural hematoma
Miscellaneous	Hydrocephalus, trauma, multiple sclerosis, epilepsy

Note. See Benson (1982) for additional etiologies.

treatable in this manner is unknown and much argued (estimates vary from 15 percent to 40 percent), but the discovery of even one individual with reversible dementia makes the study worthwhile.

CONCLUSION

This chapter has presented a scheme for the initial clinical evaluation of an individual with a dementing process. Although the scheme may appear relatively simple in outline form, the diagnostic skills demanded are considerable. Nonetheless, dementia is such a major disturbance in the lives of so many patients that the clinician must work toward a diagnosis and potential solution. By following the outline presented in this scheme, the clinician can investigate for most of the recognized causes of dementia in a systematic manner.

REFERENCES

Albert ML, Feldman RG, Willis AL: The "subcortical dementia" of progressive supranuclear palsy. J Neurol Neurosurg Psychiatry 37:121–130, 1974

Alzheimer A: A unique illness involving the cerebral cortex (translated by Hochberg CN, Hochberg FH), in Neurological Classics in Modern Translation. Edited by Rottenberg DA, Hochberg FH. New York, Hafner Press, 1977

American Psychiatric Association: Diagnostic and Statistical Manual of Mental Disorders (Third Edition). Washington, DC, American Psychiatric Association, 1980

Appell J, Kertesz A, Fisman M: A study of language functioning in Alzheimer patients. Brain Lang 17:73–91, 1982

Bayles KA: Language function in senile dementia. Brain Lang 16:265–280, 1982

Beck AT: Thinking and depression: idiosyncratic content and cognitive disorders. Arch Gen Psychiatry 9:324–333, 1963

Benson DF: The treatable dementias, in Psychiatric Aspects of Neurologic Disease (Volume 2). Edited by Benson DF, Blumer D. New York, Grune & Stratton, 1982

Benson DF: Subcortical dementia: a clinical approach, in Advances in Neurology: Volume 38. The Dementias. Edited by Mayeux R, Rosen WG. New York, Raven Press, 1983

Benson DF, Cummings JL, Tsai SY: Angular gyrus syndrome simulating Alzheimer disease. Arch Neurol 39:616–620, 1982

Benson DF, Kuhl DE, Hawkins RA, et al: The fluorodeoxyglucose ^{18}F scan in Alzheimer disease and multi-infarct dementia. Arch Neurol 40:711–714, 1983

Berg L, Danziger WL, Storandt M, et al: Predictive features in mild senile dementia of the Alzheimer type. Neurology 34:563–569, 1984

Blessed G, Tomlinson BE, Roth M: The association between quantitative measures of dementia and of senile change in the cerebral gray matter of elderly subjects. Br J Psychiatry 114:797–811, 1968

Broe GA, Akhtar AJ, Andrews GR, et al: Neurological disorders in the elderly at home. J Neurol Neurosurg Psychiat 39:362–366, 1976

Brouwers P, Cox C, Martin A, et al: Differential perceptual-spatial impairment in Huntington's and Alzheimer's patients. Arch Neurol 41:1073–1076, 1984

Brun A, Gustafson L: Limbic lobe involvement in presenile dementia. Arch Psychiat Nervenkr 226:79–93, 1978

Caine ED: Pseudodementia: current concepts and future directions. Arch Gen Psychiatry 38:1359–1364, 1981

Caplan LR, Schoene WC: Clinical features of subcortical arteriosclerotic encephalopathy (Binswanger disease). Neurology 28:1206–1215, 1978

Chase TN, Fedio P, Foster NL, et al: Wechsler Adult Intelligence Scale performance. Arch Neurol 41:1244–1247, 1984

Cummings JL: Cortical dementias, in Psychiatric Aspects of Neurologic Disease (Volume 2). Edited by Benson DF, Blumer D. New York, Grune & Stratton, 1982

Cummings JL: Organic delusions: phenomenology, anatomic correlates and review. Br J Psychiatry 146:184–197, 1985

Cummings JL, Benson DF: Dementia: a Clinical Approach. Boston, Butterworth, 1983

Cummings JL, Benson DF: Subcortical dementia. Arch Neurol 41:874–879, 1984

Cummings JL, Benson DF: Dementia of the Alzheimer type: an inventory of diagnostic clinical features. J Am Geriatr Soc 34:12–19, 1986

Cummings JL, Benson DF, Hill MA, et al: Aphasia in dementia of the Alzheimer type. Neurology 35:394–397, 1985

Cummings JL, Benson DF, LoVerme S Jr: Reversible dementia: illustrative cases, definition and review. JAMA 243:2434–2439, 1980

Cummings JL, Duchen LW: Klüver-Bucy syndrome in Pick's disease: clinical and pathologic correlations. Neurology 31:1415–1422, 1981

Davies P: Studies on the neurochemistry of central cholinergic systems in Alzheimer's disease, in Alzheimer's Disease: Senile Dementia and Related Disorders. Edited by Katzman R, Terry RD, Bick KL. New York, Raven Press, 1978

Davis PE, Mumford SJ: Cued recall and the nature of the memory disorder in dementia. Brit J Psychiat 144:383–386, 1984

De Reuck J, Crevits L. De Coster W, et al: Pathogenesis of Binswanger chronic progressive subcortical encephalopathy. Neurology 30: 920–928, 1980

Dewhurst K, Oliver J, Trick KLK, et al: Neuro-psychiatric aspects of Huntington's disease. Confini Neurologica 31:258–268, 1969

Faden AI, Townsend JJ: Myoclonus in Alzheimer disease. Arch Neurol 33:78–80, 1976

Folstein MF, Folstein SE, McHugh PR: "Mini-mental state": a practical method for grading the mental state of patients for the clinician. J. Psychiatr Res 12:189–198, 1975

Foster NL, Chase TN, Mansi L, et al: Cortical abnormalities in Alzheimer's disease. Ann Neurol 16:649–654, 1984

Groen JJ, Endtz LJ: Hereditary Pick's disease. Brain 105:443–459, 1982

Gustafson L, Hagberg B, Ingvar DH: Speech disturbances in presenile dementia related to local cerebral blood flow abnormalities in the dominant hemisphere. Brain Lang 5:103–118, 1978

Hachinski VC, Iliff LD, Zilkha E, et al: Cerebral blood flow in dementia. Arch Neurol 32:632–637, 1975

Hachinski VC, Lassen NA, Marshall J: Multi-infarct dementia: a cause of mental deterioration in the elderly. Lancet 3:207–210, 1974

Hamilton M: Development of a rating scale for primary depressive illness. British Journal of Social and Clinical Psychology 6:278–296, 1967

Hughes CP, Berg L, Danziger WL, et al: A new clinical scale for the staging of dementia. Br J Psychiatry 140:566–572, 1982

Jacob H: Muscular twitchings in Alzheimer's disease, in Alzheimer's Disease and Related Conditions. Edited by Wolstenholme GEW, O'Connor M. London, Churchill, 1970

Katzman R: The prevalence and malignancy of Alzheimer's disease. Arch Neurol 33:217–218, 1976

Katzman R, Karasu TB: The differential diagnosis of dementia, in Neurological and Sensory Disorders in the Elderly. Edited by Fields WS. New York, Grune & Stratton, 1975

Kaye DWK, Foster EM, McKechnie AA, et al: Mental illness and hospital use in the elderly: a random sample followed up. Compr Psychiatry 11:26–35, 1970

Kendell RE: The stability of psychiatric diagnoses. Br J Psychiatry 24:352–356, 1974

Kiloh LG: Pseudo-dementia. Acta Psychiatr Scand 37:336–351, 1961

Knesevich J, Martin RL, Berg L, et al: Preliminary report on affective symptoms in the early stages of senile dementia of the Alzheimer type. Am J Psychiatry 140:233–235, 1983

Koller WC, Wilson RS, Glatt SL, et al: Motor signs are infrequent in dementia of the Alzheimer type. Ann Neurol 16:514–516, 1984

Ladurner G, Iliff LD, Lechner H: Clinical factors associated with dementia in ischaemic stroke. J Neurol Neurosurg Psychiatry 45:97–101, 1982

Larssen T, Sjogren T, Jacobson G: Senile dementia: a clinical, sociomedical, and genetic study. Acta Psychiatr Scand Suppl 167:1–259, 1963

Lilly R, Cummings JL, Benson DF, et al: The human Klüver-Bucy syndrome. Neurology 33:1141–1145, 1983

Lishman WA: Organic Psychiatry. London, Blackwell Scientific, 1978

Martin A, Fedio P: Word production and comprehension in Alzheimer's disease: the breakdown of semantic knowledge. Brain Lang 19:124–141, 1983

Mayeux R, Hunter R, Fahn S: More on myoclonus in Alzheimer disease. Ann Neurol 9:200, 1981

Mayeux R, Stern Y, Rosen J, et al: Depression, intellectual impairment, and Parkinson disease. Neurology 31:645–650, 1981

McGeachie RE, Fleming JO, Shaver LR, et al: Diagnosis of Pick's disease by computed tomography. J Comput Assist Tomogr 3:113–115, 1979

McHugh PR, Folstein MF: Psychiatric syndrome of Huntington's chorea: a clinical and phenomenologic study, in Psychiatric Aspects of Neurologic Disease. Edited by Benson DF, Blumer D. New York, Grune & Stratton, 1975

McHugh PR, Folstein MF: Psychopathology of dementia: implications for neuropathology, in Congenital and Acquired Cognitive Disorders. Edited by Katzman R. New York, Raven Press, 1979

McKhann G, Drachman D, Folstein M, et al: Clinical diagnosis of Alzheimer's disease: report of the NINCDS–ADRDA Work Group under the auspices of Department of Health and Human Services Task Force on Alzheimer's Disease. Neurology 34:939–944, 1984

Miller E: On the nature of the memory disorder in presenile dementia. Neuropsychologia 9:75–81, 1971

Miller E: Efficiency of coding and the short-term memory defect in presenile dementia. Neuropsychologia 10:133–136, 1972

Nott PN, Fleminger JJ: Presenile dementia: the difficulties of early diagnosis. Acta Psychiatr Scand 51:210–217, 1975

Pearlson GD, Veroff AE, McHugh PR: The use of computed tomography in psychiatry: recent applications to schizophrenia, manic-depressive illness and dementia syndromes. Johns Hopkins Med J 149:194–202, 1981

Perez FI, Rivera VM, Meyer JS, et al: Analysis of intellectual and cognitive performance in patients with multi-infarct dementia, vertebrobasilar insufficiency with dementia, and Alzheimer's disease. J Neurol Neurosurg Psychiatr 38:533–540, 1975

Perez FI, Stump DA, Gay JRA, et al: Intellectual performance in multi-infarct dementia and Alzheimer's disease. A replication study. Can J Neurol Sci 3:181–187, 1976

Plum F: Dementia: an approaching epidemic. Nature 279:372–373, 1979

Pomara N, Reisberg B, Albers S, et al: Extrapyramidal symptoms in patients with primary degenerative dementia. J Clin Psychopharmacol 1:398–400, 1981

Post F: Dementia, depression and pseudodementia, in Psychiatric Aspects of Neurologic Disease. Edited by Benson DF, Blumer D. New York, Grune & Stratton, 1975

Reifler BV, Larson E, Hanley R: Coexistence of cognitive impairment and depression in geriatric outpatients. Am J Psychiatry 139:623–626, 1982

Robertson EE, le Roux A, Brown JH: The clinical differentiation of Pick's disease. Journal of Mental Sciences 104:1000–1024, 1958

Ron MA, Toone BK, Garralda ME, et al: Diagnostic accuracy in presenile dementia. Br J Psychiatry 134:161–168, 1979

Rosen WG, Terry RD, Fuld PA, et al: Pathological verification of ischemic score in differentiation of dementias. Ann Neurol 7:486–488, 1980

Rosenberg GA, Kornfeld M, Stovring J, et al: Subcortical arteriosclerotic encephalopathy (Binswanger): computerized tomography. Neurology 29:1102–1106, 1979

Roth M, Tomlinson BE, Blessed G: Correlation between scores for dementia and counts of "senile plaques" in cerebral gray matter of elderly subjects. Nature 209:109–110, 1966

Schlotterer G, Moscovitch M, Crapper-McLachlan D: Visual processing deficits as assessed by spatial frequency contrast sensitivity and backward masking in normal aging and Alzheimer's disease. Brain 107:309–325, 1983

Schwartz MF, Marin OSM, Saffran EM: Dissociations of language function in dementia: a case study. Brain Lang 7:277–306, 1979

Shuttleworth EC: Memory function and the clinical differentiation of dementing disorders. J Am Geriatr Soc 30:363–366, 1982

Skelton-Robinson M, Jones S: Nominal dysphasia and the severity of senile dementia. Br J Psychiatry 145:168–171, 1984

Spar JE: Dementia in the aged. Psychiatr Clin North Amer 5:67–86, 1982

Stengel E: A study of the symptomatology and differential diagnosis of Alzheimer's disease and Pick's disease. Journal of Mental Sciences 89:1–20, 1943

Storandt M, Botwinick J, Danziger WL, et al: Psychometric differentiation of mild senile dementia of the Alzheimer type. Arch Neurol 41:497–499, 1984

Sulkava R: Alzheimer's disease and senile dementia of the Alzheimer type. Acta Neurol Scand 65:636–650, 1982

Sulkava R, Haltia M, Paetau A, et al: Accuracy of clinical diagnosis in primary degenerative dementia: correlation with neuropathological findings. J Neurol Neurosurg Psychiatr 46:9–13, 1983

Tomonaga M, Yamanouchi H, Tohgi H, et al: Clinicopathologic study of progressive subcortical vascular encephalopathy (Binswanger type) in the elderly. J Am Geriatr Soc 30:524–529, 1982

Veroff AE, Pearlson GD, Ahn HS: CT scans and neuropsychological correlates of Alzheimer's disease and Huntington's disease. Brain and Cognition 1:177–184, 1982

Wechsler A, Verity M, Rosenschein S, et al: Pick's disease. Arch Neurol 39:287–290, 1982

Wells CE: Dementia: definition and description, in Dementia (2nd Edition). Edited by Wells CE. Philadelphia, Davis, 1977

Wells CE: Pseudodementia. Am J Psychiatry 136:895–900, 1979

Wells CE: Pseudodementia and the recognition of organicity, in Psychiatric Aspects of Neurologic Disease (Volume 2). Edited by Benson DF, Blumer D. New York, Grune & Stratton, 1982

Zung WWK: A self-rating depression scale. Arch Gen Psychiatry 12:63–70, 1965

2

Course of Alzheimer's Disease: A Longitudinal Study

David Shore, M.D.
Carol A. Overman, Ph.D.
Mark Tecco
Richard Jed Wyatt, M.D.

2

Course of Alzheimer's Disease: A Longitudinal Study

Alzheimer's disease (AD) is the most common dementia of later life. It is a progressive brain disorder that impairs memory and other cognitive functions. The prevalence of AD increases with age, affecting at least three percent of the population over 65 years of age. The term "Alzheimer's disease" refers to the clinical syndrome described in the *Diagnostic and Statistical Manual of Mental Disorders* (Third Edition) *(DSM-III*; American Psychiatric Association 1980) as primary degenerative dementia, of presenile or senile onset, because a diagnosis can be confirmed only by microscopic examination of brain tissue.

Recognition of the severe clinical and public health problems posed by AD has led to increased research on dementia. Results have disproven myths that attributed dementia to the normal aging process ("senility") or to arteriosclerosis. Unfortunately, there is still no satisfactory explanation of the cause of AD. Likewise, despite recent advances, there is no simple and accurate diagnostic test or generally effective treatment. To ensure that a patient is not mistakenly assumed to have AD and denied potentially effective treatment, it is essential to detect preventable or reversible (non-AD) causes of dementia. Several reviewers (Libow 1977; Wells 1978) have described clinical and laboratory evaluations that may detect causes of cognitive impairment other than AD.

There are a number of good descriptions of the clinical progression of AD symptoms (Cohen et al. 1984; Levin and Peters 1982; Mohs et al. 1982; Reisberg et al. 1984; Reisberg et al. 1982; Rosen and Mohs 1982; Semple 1982; U.S. Department of Health and Human Services 1984). In general, recent memory is the first problem area, along with visuospatial problems. Later there is confusion, disorientation, apraxia, and trouble with communication, remote memory, abstraction, and problem-solving ability. With further progression, AD patients are unable to care for themselves and are often mute or incoherent and bedridden in the final stages. Although aphasia may not be prominent until the middle to late stages of AD, some difficulty with word finding (anomia) is often evident early in its course.

In September 1984, the U. S. Department of Health and Human Services published the *Report of the Secretary's Task Force on Alzheimer's Disease*. An excerpt from the chapter on clinical course research is included here as a summary of current knowledge and promising future research directions in this area:

> Present knowledge concerning the clinical course of Alzheimer's disease is quite limited. Since early accurate diagnosis is difficult, there is relatively little information on the natural history of the disease in its early phases. Typically a patient is brought to the attention of the physician only in the later stages of the illness and in settings other than research medical centers.
>
> Knowledge about the course of Alzheimer's disease currently comes primarily from observations of clinicians and, to a lesser extent, from prospective clinical investigations. Reisberg *et al.* (1982) describe the clinical course and changes in performance on psychometric tests of patients with Alzheimer's disease. They find that initially patients complain of forgetting where they placed familiar objects and forgetting names they formerly knew well. While no objective evidence of memory impairment is apparent in the clinical interview or in social and employment situations, some psychometric indices may be found to be below average. It is extremely difficult to determine whether this represents the first stage in a progressive dementing illness or whether these symptoms represent only the manifestations of the stable "benign senescent forgetfulness" state described by Kral decades ago.
>
> Following this, clinical deficits do appear; the individual may demonstrate decreased facility in remembering names of people who have

just been introduced or may retain very little from reading a passage in a newspaper. Such persons may have no recall at all of some recent events and yet recall others well. In contrast to these lapses which occur occasionally in most people with normal mental functioning, the person with Alzheimer's disease is unable to recognize or recall even the context or related circumstances of the forgotten item or event. These difficulties become evident to intimates, and decreased performance is manifested in demanding situations at work. The patient may become seriously lost when traveling to an unfamiliar location. These symptoms are commonly accompanied by mild to moderate anxiety and by performance on psychometric tests well below average. Nevertheless, the Alzheimer's disease patient may still obtain a perfect score on the 10-item Mental Status Questionnaire.

This preliminary stage of impairment is typically followed by more serious decline. Concentration deficits can usually be elicited, and patients also display decreased knowledge of recent events, both in the context of their own personal lives and in the context of the world around them. Though patients generally have no problem traveling to familiar locations, ability to travel alone is notably curtailed, and difficulties with managing personal finances may become apparent. Complex tasks can no longer be performed accurately and efficiently. Denial is often the dominant defense mechanism at this stage, together with symptoms such as social withdrawal, flattening of affect, and loss of initiative, tact, and judgment. By this juncture, patients typically make 3 to 9 errors on the Mental Status Questionnaire; yet they may be able to function safely in a limited familiar environment with familiar routines.

In the next phase, patients can no longer survive without some assistance. They are unable, in clinical interview, to remember relevant facts regarding their own address, or phone number, or the names of close family members, of their high school or college, though they invariably know their own names and those of their spouse and children. Toileting and eating activities remain intact, though difficulty in selecting the proper clothing to wear is a common problem. Even in this phase, there may be episodes of lucidity.

As the disease progresses, patients may occasionally forget the name of their spouse and become largely unaware of all recent events and experiences in their lives. Typically, they are by now unaware of their surroundings, the year, or the season. Diurnal rhythm frequently becomes disturbed, and episodes of incontinence may appear. Personality and emotional changes often manifest themselves and are quite variable, often including delusional and paranoid behavior, such as accusing a spouse of being an imposter, or talking to imaginary figures in the environment; obsessive symptoms, such as repetitive washing of the dishes; anxiety symptoms, agitation, and newly manifested violent and abusive behavior; and an inability to act because of the inability to retain a thought long enough to pursue a purposeful course of action. The changes just described—particularly the inability to recognize a spouse or other caregiver, incontinence, and/or emotional outbursts—are especially difficult burdens for the caring family members and are often the reasons for seeking institutional care for the patient.

Ultimately, all verbal abilities are lost; the patient is incontinent of urine, requires assistance in toileting and eating, and may lose the ability to walk. At late stages of the disease, generalized cortical, as well as focal neurologic, signs and symptoms are frequently present. Invariably, patients with late dementia make 10 errors on the Mental Status Questionnaire.

Although the above observations are exceedingly rich clinically and provide a useful starting point for further research, nevertheless many important issues relating to clinical course remain unexamined. There is a general consensus about the latest phases of Alzheimer's disease, and there is a reasonable degree of agreement about the approximate sequence of intermediate deficits. However, there is still great difficulty recognizing the disease in the early stages. Little attention has been paid in the research literature to the enormous variability in rate of deterioration and the vast differences in duration of disease—from 2 to 20 years. Investigators have often failed to control for confounding factors such as years of education, general physical health, premorbid personality features, family and informal supports, and capacity for self-care. Few longitudinal studies of the course of illness have been carried out, family history is commonly not included in research designs, and individual differences are often overlooked.

Typically, performance on diagnostic screening instruments and pyschometric tests has not been especially well correlated with actual capacity for self-care and for life in the community. What intervening factors might be responsible for shaping, hastening, or delaying the inevitable progression of symptomatology? . . . Can measures be developed that will accurately predict when a given symptom will occur in a given patient, beyond assuming that cognitive deterioration will progress? While certain core symptoms such as difficulty with new learning; disorientation for time, place, and person; apraxia; and ultimately, aphasia are often cited as hallmarks of Alzheimer's dementia, secondary psychiatric symptoms are far less predictable in nature and often pose far greater burdens for the caregiver.

Finally, in terms of systematic longitudinal research, which tests are most useful for sensitively monitoring the increasing rates and

> severity of deterioration in Alzheimer's disease? Hersch's Extended Scale for Dementia and Reisberg's Global Deterioration Scale for Assessment of Primary Degenerative Dementia appear to be useful measures in documenting the progressive global decline in cognition, behavior, and affect in Alzheimer's disease patients. However, the development of more sensitive and specific biological and behavioral measures is urgently needed. (U.S. Department of Health and Human Services 1984, pp 29–33)

As this excerpt indicates, the progression of AD needs to be studied and documented. Although AD has been described as a diagnosis of exclusion, it is important to note that the *DSM–III* diagnostic criteria require the dementia to have an "insidious onset with uniformly progressive deteriorating course" (p 126). A number of cognitive tests have been used to screen for dementia of the Alzheimer type, but few have been useful in objective documentation of deterioration over time. Because the rate of decline varies from patient to patient, and may vary over time in a given patient, we have sought to determine whether certain objective cognitive and language tests might show significant decline over different periods of time in patients meeting AD symptom and course diagnostic criteria.

METHODS

At the National Institute of Mental Health, we conducted a longitudinal study of AD outpatients. Patients diagnosed by private psychiatrists and neurologists as having early AD were referred for potential participation in this study. Some families learned of the study through local chapters of the Alzheimer's Disease and Related Disorders Association. If prospective research patients had the ability to take simple verbal and written tests and wished to enter the protocol, we first reviewed their general medical, neurologic, and psychiatric workups. In-person evaluations were scheduled for those AD patients without significant hypertension or unstable medical problems. Informed consent was obtained from patients and their legally authorized representatives after explanation of the protocol.

Our evaluations consisted of physical and neurologic examinations; blood studies; and vision, hearing, and speech (language/aphasia) tests. Only those patients scoring below 6 on the Hachinski Ischemic Scale (Hachinski 1978) were accepted into the study. In general, the higher the Hachinski score, the more likely it is that symptoms of cognitive deficit are due to multiinfarct (rather than AD-type) dementia. Although we were unable to exclude all patients taking medications, we attempted to keep medication dosages as stable as possible throughout the study. The protocol involved administration of placebo and sodium fluoride in a double-blind ABA crossover design. Rationale for this trial and methodologic considerations have been described elsewhere (Shore and Wyatt 1982, 1983). Because sodium fluoride has no known psychotropic effects at the dosage range used here and did not have any significant effect on the course of AD during this study, we evaluated the data collected during a two-year period regardless of fluoride or placebo administration.

All AD patients were tested using the Extended Scale for Dementia (ESD) (Hersch 1979), the Mini-Mental Status (MMS) examination (Folstein, Folstein, and McHugh 1975), the Mental Status Questionnaire (MSQ) (Brink et al. 1978), and the Porch Index of Communicative Ability (PICA) (Porch 1971).

The ESD is an objective test (similar to the Mattis Dementia Scale; Mattis 1976) of a wide variety of cognitive functions. The ESD questions are generally "easy" for normal elderly subjects, and the test can be given in less than one hour, yielding a score of up to 250 points. Well-educated, age-matched normal controls (spouses of our AD outpatients) generally scored between 240 and 250 on this scale. The ESD has been validated (Hersch 1979), and significant declines have been found in the scores of AD patients tested at six-month intervals.

The PICA is a test of speech and language abilities administered by a speech pathologist trained in its usage. This test can be given in less than one hour and provides scores on gestural, verbal, and graphomotor subscales, as well as an overall average (OA). Scores range from 0 to 15. All of the age-matched controls scored an OA higher than 14.30 on the PICA.

Most MSQ questions deal with orientation and general information; scores range from 0 to 10 (Brink et al. 1978). Our age-matched controls scored 10 correct on the MSQ. MMS questions cover orientation, registration, attention and calculations, recall, and language areas; scores range from 0 to 30 (Folstein et al. 1975).

Six AD patients took the ESD, MMS, MSQ, and PICA at three-month intervals for two years. These patients initially were mildly to moderately demented and were brought by their families for the follow-up tests. The healthy spouses of these AD patients took these same tests during the initial evaluation and yearly thereafter. The tests described previously were given by the same person throughout the study. The patients' average age was 63.5 years; the spouses' average age was 63.3 years.

To determine which tests were able to detect significant declines in scores over various periods of time (six months to two years), Wilcoxon matched-pairs signed-ranks tests were used.

RESULTS

Mean ($\pm$ standard deviation) baseline one- and two-year follow-up test scores of the AD patients are shown in Table 1. The ESD scores showed significant deterioration in the AD patients for each of the two 12-month intervals ($Z = -2.20$, $p = .028$ for first year; $Z = -1.99$, $p = .046$ for second year). Because the ESD was designed to show cognitive decline in dementia patients over time, this result was expected. The MMS scores of the AD patients showed a significant decline during the second year ($Z = -1.99$,

Table 1. Baseline and Follow-Up Test Scores of Alzheimer's Disease Patients ($N = 6$)

	Baseline		One-Year Follow-up		Two-Year Follow-up	
Test	*M*	*SD*	*M*	*SD*	*M*	*SD*
Extended Scale for Dementia	169.8	41.1	141.8	54.2	101.7	35.5
Overall Average Porch Index of Communicative Ability	12.03	1.95	9.15	4.68	8.03	1.87
Mini-Mental Status	19.2	6.8	18.0	6.3	10.2	5.2
Mental Status Questionnaire	6.8	2.1	5.7	2.6	3.0	1.9

$p = .046$) but not the first. The AD patients' MSQ results showed nonsignificant trends for declining scores during each of the two years of follow-up. There were significant declines from baseline at the 24-month follow-up testing of the AD patients for both the MMS and the MSQ ($Z = -2.20$, $p = .028$ for both). The AD patients' OA PICA scores showed a significant decline during the first year of follow-up ($Z = -2.20$, $p = .028$) but not the second.

The age-matched controls (the spouses) showed no decline in scores on any of the tests when retested after a one-year interval (see Table 2). The AD patient's baseline scores on the ESD, OA PICA, MMS, and MSQ were lower than those of the healthy spouse in every case. In fact, the lowest scores on these tests among the controls were higher than the highest scores of any AD patient during the study. Two of the AD patients had MMS scores of 25, and 4 had MSQ scores of 8 or 9 during the first year of testing.

DISCUSSION

As noted in a previous report (Shore et al. 1983), some of our patients showed improvements in ESD and other test scores at the first or second retesting session. When first brought in for testing, some AD patients seemed anxious about facing new people in a new environment. After two or more visits, these patients appeared more calm and secure; they recognized the faces of our staff and seemed to know that they would not be mistreated (although they had trouble remembering our names or which questions

Table 2. Baseline and One-Year Follow-Up Test Scores of Spouses of Patients With Alzheimer's Disease ($N = 6$)

	Baseline		One-Year Follow-up	
Test	*M*	*SD*	*M*	*SD*
Extended Scale for Dementia	246.5	2.5	247.9	2.1
Overall Average Porch Index of Communicative Ability	14.80	0.19	14.77	0.12
Mini-Mental Status	29.3	0.5	28.8	1.0
Mental Status Questionnaire	10.0	0.0	10.0	0.0

they had been asked). We suggest that for some patients the first day's test results may be artifactually low. This seems to be more common among the better functioning patients: Two of the 4 patients with initial ESD scores above 180 had the same or higher scores on the first retesting. None of the patients who started below 180 improved at the first (three-month) follow-up visit.

One patient was initially accepted into the study, but his data are not presented because he did not show the clinical deterioration required to diagnose AD. His initial MMS score was 24; MSQ, 8; ESD, 192; and OA PICA, 13.85. None of these scores decreased, even after two years of testing, consistent with other elderly subjects having less severe, nonprogressive cognitive problems as described by Reisberg et al. (1982, 1984).

Very few patients, even early in the course of AD, could complete detailed self-rating forms. Patients seemed to have difficulty remembering the instructions, and their method of responding sometimes changed from page to page. Some patients checked the same box for all the questions on a given page. Whereas several patients who scored above 180 on the ESD could adequately complete the Inventory of Psychic and Somatic Complaints–Elderly (IPSC–E) by themselves, none of those patients who scored below 150 (ESD) could do so.

All of the spouses (or other immediate family) noted the AD patients' progressive deterioration in memory, communication, self-care, and so on during the two years of follow-up. A few spouses felt that the decline was more rapid during some months than others, or that the patients seemed to have "some good days and some bad days." None, however, noted extreme variability (except perhaps for secondary symptoms like agitation) or any lasting and meaningful improvement in cognitive or self-care abilities.

The lack of change in test scores of the healthy spouses after an interval of one year was expected because the tests were not designed to demonstrate the more subtle changes of normal aging. The tests we used were simple and, except for the PICA, not timed. (Other studies have shown that speed and performance on complex new tasks may be impaired with normal aging.)

In many cases, a clinical diagnosis of Alzheimer's disease (AD) is made during a one-time (cross-sectional) evaluation. Because DSM III diagnostic criteria for primary degenerative dementia (referred to here as AD) require a dementia with insidious onset and progressive deteriorating course, a longitudinal evaluation of dementia is preferable. A number of reports have concluded that many patients diagnosed as having a progressive dementia do not show the expected course and outcome. Examples of such studies are described by Garcia et al. (1981) and Shore et al. (1983). The former authors noted that several long-term follow-up studies of patients diagnosed as having dementia showed that 11 percent to 57 percent of such patients proved not to be demented. The source of error in such cases is considered to reflect current limitations of neuropsychiatric diagnosis. Following the patient's clinical course greatly improves accuracy of the diagnosis (Garcia et al. 1981). Although more recently Reding et al. (1984) described an improvement in the ability to predict progressive dementia, this was accomplished at a special dementia research center using review of medical records, comprehensive laboratory and radiographic studies, and a series of neuropsychologic tests.

We previously (Shore et al. 1983) noted the importance of cognitive testing to help separate subjective from objective deficits and to establish a baseline for documenting deterioration over time. Many elderly people with very mild impairments on testing, including those with a slight or mild degree of atrophy on computed tomographic (CT) scans, do not show the clinical course of AD. As Reisberg et al. (1984) noted, forgetfulness to a less disabling degree is common in the elderly and often is not progressive in nature. Some older people may have to take early retirement from their jobs because of difficulty in carrying out their work responsibilities without necessarily having the course and outcome expected in AD.

Many people over 65 years of age have a subjective sense that their memory is not as good as it was when they were younger; however, they do not generally show the deterioration typical of AD during a follow-up period of greater than two years (Reisberg et al. 1984). Only when patients had decreased ability to manage money, do shopping, and so on did they commonly have subsequent clinical deterioration typical of AD (Reisberg et al. 1982, 1984). At this stage, patients frequently make three or more errors on the MSQ, although they may be oriented, recognize familiar people and faces, and travel to familiar places. Such studies may be valuable in separating patients with benign senescent forgetfulness from those with AD.

We have considered the possibility that some patients who seem to have long "plateau" periods in the course of a dementia may in fact have two separate conditions. That is, a person may experience some forgetfulness around 60 years of age, show no deterioration during the next 10 years, and then independently develop AD with its progressive deteriorating course. In elderly patients with benign forgetfulness, results of MSQ or MMS tests may indicate mild impairment. This may be indistinguishable from that of patients in the earliest stages of AD. Until we have reliable tests that can separate the two (as discussed in the next section), repeated testing over time is strongly advised.

The data reported in this paper suggest that the ESD can demonstrate significant deterioration during each of two successive 12-month follow-up intervals in a small group of patients with AD. The OA PICA, a test of language and communication skills, showed significant deterioration during the first but not the second year of follow-up. It may be more sensitive to change earlier in the course of AD.

The OA PICA results are quite different from those seen with the MMS, which showed significant deterioration during the second but not the first year of follow-up. Because many patients become quite confused and disoriented during the middle rather than the earlier stages of AD, this result was not unexpected. The MSQ scores decreased significantly during the 24-month interval only, not during either 12-month interval.

The present results need to be replicated and extended in larger samples. We are encouraged by the ability of the ESD to document cognitive decline in AD patients over long periods of time and hope that other instruments can be developed to objectively monitor cognitive deterioration throughout the course of AD.

SUGGESTIONS FOR FUTURE STUDIES

Clearly, it would be most advantageous to distinguish as early as possible those elderly persons who will have the progressive deteriorating course of AD from those who will have a relatively benign prognosis. One test that may be useful in this regard involves visuospatial tasks, such as the ability to draw in the numbers and hands on a circle to show a clock face at a particular hour. Elderly persons with a benign form of forgetfulness may perform this type of visuospatial task rather easily, whereas those with early AD may have great difficulty carrying out this task. This type of task needs to be quantified and tested in the future to determine whether it has genuine prognostic value.

Another test that may help distinguish early AD patients from depressed and other elderly patients was described by Weingartner and Silberman (1982). They noted that the relational properties of words in a list typically facilitate recall of such words by depressed patients and normal controls. Patients with AD, however, cannot learn and recall inherently organized information (for example, words related by a category such as "vegetables") any better than unrelated words in a list. Again, future research may clarify the potential value of such assessments.

SUMMARY AND CONCLUSIONS

There are many good clinical descriptions of the typical clinical decline of AD patients (Cohen et al. 1984; Levin and Peters 1982; Mohs et al. 1982; Reisberg et al. 1982; Rosen and Mohs 1982; Semple et al. 1982; U. S. Department of Health and Human Services 1984), but few have objectively documented the decline in longitudinal fashion. We believe that tests like the ESD can be useful in documenting the diagnosis, course, and possible treatment response of AD patients. Because there is no clinically useful treatment generally available for AD patients at this time, repeated testing may be helpful in detecting patients whose cognitive impairments do not worsen. This would suggest that a pseudodementia or non-AD dementia, perhaps more treatable, might be present. Such testing should be done by the same person, in the same place, several times over a period of at least a year.

We think it is also worth noting that even relatively early in the course of AD, the OA PICA revealed some difficulty with language. Some of these patients did not have clinically apparent aphasia, except for occasional word-finding problems, but repeated testing revealed progressive impairment during the first year of follow-up.

References

American Psychiatric Association. Diagnostic and Statistical Manual of Mental Disorders (Third Edition). Washington, DC, American Psychiatric Association, 1980

Brink TL, Capri D, DeNeeve V, et al: Senile confusion: limitations of assessment by the face-hand test, mental status questionnaire, and staff ratings. J Am Geriatr Soc 26:380–382, 1978

Cohen D, Kennedy G, Eisdorfer C: Phases of change in the patient with Alzheimer's dementia; a conceptual dimension for defining health care management. J Am Geriatr Soc 32:11–15, 1984

Folstein MF, Folstein SE, McHugh PR: "Mini-Mental State": a practical method for grading the cognitive state of patients for the clinician. J Psychiatr Res 12:189–198, 1975

Garcia CA, Reding MJ, Blass JP: Overdiagnosis of dementia. J Am Geriatr Soc 29:407–410, 1981

Hachinski V: Cerebral blood flow: differentiation of Alzheimer's disease from multi-infarct dementia, in Alzheimer's Disease: Senile Dementia and Related Disorders. Edited by Katzman R, Terry RD, Bick KL, New York, Raven Press, 1978

Hersch EL: Development and application of the extended scale for dementia. J Am Geriatr Soc 27:348–354, 1979

Levin HS, Peters BH: Report of the ad hoc committee for the classification of the severity of Alzheimer's disease, in Alzheimer's Disease: A Report of Progress. Edited by Corkin S, Growden JH, Davis KL, et al. New York, Raven Press, 1982

Libow L: Senile dementia and "pseudosenility": clinical diagnosis, in Cognitive and Emotional Disturbance in the Elderly. Edited by Eisdorfer C, Friedel RO. Chicago, Year Book Medical Publishing, 1977

Mattis S: Dementia rating scale, in Geriatric Psychiatry. Edited by Bellak R, Karasu B. New York, Grune and Stratton, 1976

Mohs RC, Rosen WG, Davis KL: Defining treatment efficacy in patients with Alzheimer's disease, in Alzheimer's Disease: A Report of Progress. Edited by Corkin S, Growden JH, Davis KL, et al. New York, Raven Press, 1982

Porch BE: Porch index of communicative ability. Palo Alto, CA, Consulting Psychologists Press, 1971

Reding MJ, Haycox J, Wigforss K, et al: Follow-up of patients referred to a dementia service. J Am Geriatr Soc 32:265–268, 1984

Reisberg B, Ferris S, Anand R, et al: Clinical assessments of cognition in the aged, in Dementia in the Elderly. Edited by Shamoian, CA. Washington, DC, American Psychiatric Press, 1984

Reisberg B, Ferris SH, Crook T: Signs, symptoms, and course of age-associated cognitive decline, in Alzheimer's Disease: A Report of Progress. Edited by Corkin S, Growden JH, Davis KL, et al. New York, Raven Press, 1982

Rosen WG, Mohs RC: Evolution of cognitive decline in dementia, in Alzheimer's Disease: A Report of Progress. Edited by Corkin S, Growden JH, Davis KL, et al. New York, Raven Press, 1982

Semple SA, Smith CM, Swash M: The Alzheimer disease syndrome, in Alzheimer's Disease: A Report of Progress. Edited by Corkin S, Growden JH, Davis KL, et al. New York, Raven Press, 1982

Shore D, Overman CA, Wyatt RJ: Improving diagnostic accuracy in the diagnosis of Alzheimer's disease. J Clin Psychiatry 44:207–212, 1983

Shore D, Wyatt RJ: Research design issues: antialuminum drug studies in Alzheimer's disease. Clin Neuropharmacol 5:337–343, 1982

Shore D, Wyatt RJ: Aluminum and Alzheimer's disease. J Nerv Ment Dis 171:553–558, 1983

U. S. Department of Health and Human Services: Alzheimer's Disease—Report of the Secretary's Task Force on Alzheimer's Disease. Washington, DC, U.S. Government Printing Office, 1984

Weingartner H, Silberman E: Models of cognitive impairment: cognitive changes in depression. Psychopharmacol Bull 18:27–42, 1982

Wells CE: Chronic brain disease: an overview. Am J Psychiatry 135:1–12, 1978

3

Schizophrenic Dementia

Karen Faith Berman, M.D.
Daniel R. Weinberger, M.D.

3

Schizophrenic Dementia

The question of whether schizophrenia is an organic disease with underlying physical brain pathology has held a prominent place in the interest of researchers and clinicians in psychiatry for as long as this illness has been studied. A great deal of speculation and research has been directed toward delineating the nature of the putative physical lesion and its clinical concomitants. In particular, theoreticians, researchers, and clinicians have pondered whether schizophrenia may be characterized or accompanied by dementia.

Kraepelin's view of schizophrenia as a precocious dementia is supported by recent research findings indicating that a true dementia with underlying neuropathologic factors and impaired physiologic processes is central to this illness. Many of the clinical symptoms of schizophrenia (for example flat affect, poor insight, diminished motivation, poor social judgment, impaired goal-oriented behavior, and lack of appropriate concern for personal hygiene) are similar to those seen in organic dementia. Features such as peculiarities of gait and posture, disordered smooth-pursuit eye movements, minor ("soft") neurologic signs, and electroen-

---

This chapter was written by the authors in their personal capacity and does not necessarily reflect the views of the National Institute of Mental Health.

cephalographic abnormalities further suggest a link between schizophrenia and central nervous system pathology. More conclusive evidence is offered by neuropsychologic, neuroradiologic, and neurophysiologic studies, some of which are reviewed in this chapter. Despite this growing body of evidence, the concept of a schizophrenic dementia remains controversial.

A number of factors have hampered attempts to definitively resolve this important question. Foremost among these have been 1) inconsistent nomenclature and lack of standardized or useful diagnostic criteria, and 2) limitations in the methodologies available for studying the structure and function of the human brain in living subjects. Because a great deal of progress has been made in both these arenas over the last decade, a reassessment of the notion of "schizophrenic dementia" is timely. This issue has great potential impact on future directions to be taken by research and treatment and is, therefore, quite important.

In this chapter we consider recent developments in the diagnosis approach to schizophrenia that have direct implications for the concept of schizophrenic dementia. We discuss new techniques for in vivo measurement of brain structure and function that have been brought to bear on the question of neurostructural and neurophysiologic concomitants of this illness and, when used in conjunction with neuropsychological studies, may provide incisive indicators of brain status. Next, we review the findings of such studies, and these data are synthesized into a proposed framework for conceptualizing schizophrenic dementia.

HISTORY AND BACKGROUND

Toward the end of the 19th century, in what are now considered classic studies and papers, the German psychiatrist Emil Kraepelin (1919) laid the groundwork for many of the present views of schizophrenia. He noted that whereas some mentally ill patients with psychosis achieved full recovery of their premorbid personalities and intellectual capacities, others exhibited progressive functional impairment leading to a cognitively deteriorated state with many features of a dementia. In his 1896 *Textbook of Psychiatry*,

Kraepelin differentiated the "functional psychoses" into two diagnostic entities based on course and outcome. Although he referred to the illness of patients who fully reconstituted as *manic depressive psychosis*, he used the term *dementia praecox* to describe the syndrome of those with poor prognosis and chronic course. His choice of the latter term was based upon his observation of clinical similarities between patients with dementia praecox and those with known neurologic disorders such as epilepsy, encephalitis, and general paresis.

Despite his early emphasis on the chronic unremitting nature and poor outcome of these "deteriorating psychoses," Kraepelin at one point included in the diagnostic category of dementia praecox patients having clinical signs and symptoms of psychosis but not having chronic course and intellectual deterioration. In 1911 Kraepelin's Swiss colleague Eugen Bleuler (1950) further embraced this liberal stance and offered a broader approach to the diagnosis and conceptualization of schizophrenia (as well as the name "schizophrenia" itself). Bleuler, too, believed that patients with schizophrenia never regained full premorbid function (*restitutio ad integrum*). However, in formulating diagnoses he placed more emphasis on the presence of what he considered to be specific psychopathologic reactions, "splitting" of psychic functions, and consequent "divorce from reality," rather than on unremitting course and poor outcome.

This trend toward diagnosing solely on the basis of poorly defined and unspecified symptoms such as those proposed by Bleuler, without regard to course of the illness, came to be widely accepted during the first part of the 20th century. Unfortunately, this set the stage for a great deal of nosologic confusion. The diagnostic dilemma climaxed in the 1950s and 1960s, when emphasis on the cross-sectional clinical picture (rather than on the course of the illness) dovetailed with psychiatrists' tendency to be more concerned with social and psychologic factors in schizophrenia. In this process, concepts of cognitive deficit, deterioration, and dementia in schizophrenia languished. In fact, the first and second editions of the *Diagnostic and Statistical Manual of Mental Disorders* (American Psychiatric Association 1952, 1965) as well as many textbooks (for example, Kaplan et al. 1980) tended to minimize or entirely overlook the occurrence of cognitive deficits suggestive of dementia in patients with schizophrenia.

Nonetheless, since the time of Kraepelin and regardless of the current diagnostic dogma that prevailed, experienced clinicians have continued to note that a proportion of patients with schizophrenia do have a deteriorating course ultimately resulting in a "defect state" with diminished intellectual function. Zubin et al. (1980) suggested that 10 percent of patients with schizophrenia have a chronic course ending in severe dementia. Likewise, neuropsychometric studies have repeatedly and consistently documented that schizophrenic patients perform poorly on a variety of cognitive tests. Perhaps in response to these observations, the third edition of the *Diagnostic and Statistical Manual of Mental Disorders* (*DSM–III;* American Psychiatric Association 1980) addresses the possibility of dementia in schizophrenia. For example, with regard to differential diagnosis between the two, these diacritic guidelines are offered: "Schizophrenia, especially when chronic, may be associated with some degree of intellectual deterioration" (p 110) and "it is possible for an individual with schizophrenia to have superimposed organic mental disorder" (p 186).

Thus, according to the current diagnostic schema, the diagnoses of dementia and schizophrenia are no longer mutually exclusive. In this effort to reflect more closely the clinical and neuropsychometric data available to us and to delineate specific and meaningful diagnostic criteria that have prognostic value and implications for treatment, *DSM–III* represents an improvement over many previous proposals.

Any real heuristic gain that might evolve from *DSM–III* remains limited as long as causative factors and physical concomitants of schizophrenia remain unknown and "construct validity" for diagnostic criteria remains unproven. Construct validity refers to the ability to independently corroborate derived data (such as diagnoses of schizophrenia) using other, independent sources (such as pathognomonic laboratory tests) (Mosher 1980). Although we clearly have no laboratory tests to confirm diagnoses of schizophrenia, a full spectrum of techniques are now available for assessing brain status, ranging from time-honored clinical measures of phenomenology and neuropsychologic function to highly sensitive and technical innovations that probe actual structure and function in the living human brain. Correlative, cross-modal studies carried out using, in various combinations, the full panoply of tools can help to validate hypotheses about schizophrenia and refine its working definition. As discussed later, the investigation of cognitive function and intellectual capacity in schizophrenia offers an excellent opportunity to apply this multimodal approach.

COGNITIVE AND INTELLECTUAL FUNCTION IN SCHIZOPHRENIA

Several excellent reports have summarized the extensive literature comparing cognitive and perceptual testing (of intelligence, visuospatial ability, visual memory, concept formation, motor speed, and problem-solving abilities) in schizophrenia with that of other psychiatric or brain-damaged patients (Goldstein 1978; Heaton et al. 1978; Malec 1978). Although many of the studies reviewed were criticized on the basis of methodologic limitations (including nonstandardized diagnostic criteria and poor control for age, IQ, education, length of hospitalization, and medication effects), consistent findings were noted. In most studies, cognitive deficits were demonstrated in patients with schizophrenia, especially those who were chronic, when compared with normative values or with other nonorganic psychiatric groups (Heaton et al. 1978). Heaton and colleagues reviewed 94 studies published between 1965 and 1978 and found that nonpsychotic mentally disordered patients could be reliably discriminated from those with known organic disease with 82 percent accuracy. In contrast, patients with chronic schizophrenia were distinguished from brain-damaged controls at an essentially chance rate of 54 percent. These reviewers suggested that patients with chronic schizophrenia have a cerebral deficit, because they perform similarly to diffusely brain-damaged patients and cannot be statistically differentiated from them.

A number of investigators (for example, DeWolfe et al. 1971; Goldstein and Halperin 1977; Klonoff et al. 1970) studied chronic patients using the Halstead-Reitan Battery, a set of tests sensitive to cerebral dysfunction. Almost all individual tests in this extensive battery as well as the Average Impairment Index, a summary score of performance on the battery, were markedly abnormal. The impairment index correlated with low IQ and higher medication dosage in Klonoff's study, and Goldstein and Halperin found that patients with long-term hospitalization and nonparanoid clinical pictures were most impaired on neuropsychologic tests. The latter finding raises the question of the role of psychotic symptoms in neuropsychometric deficits as well as the possibility that these cognitive deficits may comprise or be associated with defect symptoms.

Some studies have documented that patients with productive symptoms such as hallucinations, delusions, bizarre or inappropriate affect, and thought disorder are less impaired than patients with predominantly defect symptoms such as flat affect, mutism, withdrawal, and apathy. Lilliston (1973), for example, found that subjects with no cognitive deficits on visuospatial tests were anxious and tended to overreact to stimuli, whereas those whose test results indicated a "high probability of cerebral damage" were characterized by withdrawal, apathy, and little affect. This has suggested to some (for example, Seidman 1983) that preoccupation with florid psychotic symptoms is not a viable explanation for the poor cognitive test performance of patients with chronic schizophrenia as a whole.

With regard to the course of schizophrenic dementia, several longitudinal studies (for example, Haywood and Moelis 1963) found little evidence of general intellectual decline after the acute onset of the disorder in patients who improved clinically, but they noted that clinically unimproved patients deteriorated somewhat in overall IQ. Smith (1964) reported that 17 patients who were followed for eight years showed no deterioration on most measures. Interestingly, however, 10 of these subjects did manifest a specific deterioration on a Weigl-type set-shifting test. This fact is especially intriguing because deficits on the Wisconsin Card Sort, a currently used version, have been shown to be extremely sensitive indicators of the integrity of the frontal cortex in humans (Milner 1963, 1964, 1971; Milner and Petrides 1984) and of damage to dorsolateral prefrontal cortex (DLPFC) in particular.

Poor performance on the Wisconsin Card Sort has also proved to be one of the most consistent and reliable findings in schizophrenia (Kolb and Whishaw 1983; Malmo 1974). Kolb and Whishaw administered to patients with schizophrenia a battery of tests selectively sensitive to left or right frontal, temporal, or parietal function. Patients were particularly impaired on tests of right and left frontal lobes. Pronounced psychomotor deficits on tasks requiring continuous processing of sequential or spatially peripheral stimuli have been interpreted as further evidence of frontal lobe impairment in this illness (Levin 1984).

Clearly, there is no paucity of studies of cognition in schizophrenia. However, this seemingly extensive and relatively consistent literature on the subject has not resolved the controversy surrounding the concept of cognitive deficits in schizophrenia. That deficits have been observed to various degrees on almost all tasks administered has led some schizophrenia researchers to conclude that these impairments are not only nonspecific but may reflect purely psychological (for example, attentional and motivational) problems. Others suggested that cognitive impairments in schizophrenia reflect the effects of institutionalization and treatment rather than a dementia associated with the disorder itself (Jellinek 1976; Marsden 1976). Similarly, the fact that a given subject may perform better at some times than at others, has suggested to some investigators that patients perform poorly on these assessments because they are unwilling rather than unable to perform, or that if they are unable such inability is secondary to ongoing psychosis. Past failures of the research community to ascertain and demonstrate consistent biological underpinnings of these cognitive disabilities have bolstered these opinions.

The opposing view—that some patients score in the "organic" range on these tests because they do, indeed, have underlying organic pathology—has, until relatively recently, been extremely difficult to support. More sophisticated neuroradiologic techniques, in particular x-ray computed tomographic (CT) scanning, have given this field a new perspective and lent new credence to the concept of a schizophrenic dementia. The *DSM–III* suggests that when schizophrenia is "associated with some degree of intellectual deterioration, [the] absence of identifiable brain pathology helps rule out the additional diagnosis of dementia" (p 110). However, establishing the presence or "absence of identifiable brain pathology," as suggested, is a relative concept that has been revolutionized by new brain-imaging techniques.

CORRELATIONS BETWEEN CT FINDINGS AND COGNITIVE FUNCTION

In most of the more than 30 controlled studies using CT to delineate brain structure in schizophrenia, some percentage of patients investigated has been found to have abnormalities (Weinberger 1984). Although the data put forth in these studies are not entirely consistent, some of the primary findings have withstood the tests of time and replication and have, in fact, been supported by almost all relevant investigations. The most prevalent and consistent findings in patients are enlarged cerebral ventricles, signs of cortical atrophy, or both. Atrophy of the cerebellar vermis (Weinberger 1984), changes in radiodensity of brain parenchyma (Dewan et al. 1983; Golden et al. 1981), and reversals of normal hemispheric asymmetries (Luchins et al. 1982) have also been described. One recent study reports that cortical atrophy is most common in frontal cortex (Shelton et al. 1985). Although no single finding is pathognomonic of schizophrenia, and, indeed, most patients have no grossly demonstrable CT findings, it is clear that neurostructural abnormalities suggestive of an underlying neuropathologic process occur more frequently in patients with schizophrenia than in normal individuals (Weinberger et al. 1983).

A number of reports have further suggested that the degree to which these CT indicators of brain pathology are present in a given patient and the degree to which that patient is cognitively impaired are positively related (Zec and Weinberger, 1986). This lends credence, on the one hand, to the notion that the cognitive and intellectual deficits have an organic basis and, on the other hand, to the idea that such structural abnormalities have clinical and heuristic meaning in schizophrenia.

In Table 1 selected studies that have explored cognitive function and brain structure are summarized. The earliest report (Haug 1962) showed a strong relationship between degree of dementia (defined by subjective evaluation of intellectual and psychosocial deterioration) and ventricular enlargement on pneumoencephalography in 101 schizophrenic patients.

Johnstone et al. (1976, 1978) studied 18 patients (mean age, 58 years) who were hospitalized for an average of 32 years and diagnosed as having chronic schizophrenia as defined by Feighner criteria (Feighner et al. 1972). Johnstone and colleagues reported a correlation between ventricular size and cognitive deficit as determined by performance on the Withers and Hinton Mental Status Exam, a somewhat limited screening tool. Impairment was especially noted on serial 7s and delayed-recall memory items. Several other CT studies suggest a relationship between brain structure and performance on the Withers and Hinton battery. However, the implied relationship was not always linear (Owens et al. 1985), and in one study (Famuyiwa et al. 1979) it was only apparent after the exclusion of patients with tardive dyskinesia.

In several studies Golden et al. (1980a, 1980b, 1982) investigated cognition using the Luria-Nebraska Neuropsychological Battery, an extensive exam with 14 subscales that takes several hours to complete. Although idiosyncratic methods for evaluating CT scans may have been used, the combined sample of these studies probably represents the largest series of patients reported for whom CT scans and comprehensive neuropsychological evaluations are available. Many of the subscale scores were found to correlate with CT findings, and the scores were to an appreciable degree predictive of CT abnormalities.

Findings on the Halstead-Reitan Neuropsychological Battery and the Wechsler Adult Intelligence Scale have also been compared with CT scans. In general, performance IQ was lower in patients with large cerebral ventricles (Lawson et al. in press) and

Table 1. Selected Studies of Structural Brain Abnormalities and Clinical Correlates in Schizophrenia

Study	Subjects	Abnormal structure measure	Clinical correlates
Haug (1962)	101 schizophrenics	Ventricular size (pneumoenceph-alography)	Intellectual and psycho-social deterioration
Holden et al. (1973)	65 schizophrenics	Third ventricle (echoenceph-alography)	Treatment resistance
Johnstone et al. (1976)	18 schizophrenics	Lateral ventricular size (CT)	Intellectual impairment (Withers and Hinton test)
Johnstone et al. (1978)	18 schizophrenics; 10 medical controls	Lateral ventricular size (CT)	Intellectual impairment (Withers and Hinton test), negative symp-toms
Famuyiwa et al. (1979)	45 schizophrenics	Ventricular enlarge-ment (CT)	Paired associative learn-ing (only patients with no tardive dyskinesia)
Reider et al. (1979)	17 schizophrenics	Sulcal prominence (CT)	Intellectual impairment (Halstead-Reitan Neuropsychological Battery)
Donnelly et al. (1980)	15 schizophrenics	Lateral ventricular size (CT)	Intellectual impairment (Halstead-Reitan Neuropsychological Battery)
Golden et al. (1980)	42 schizophrenics	Lateral ventricular size (CT)	Intellectual impairment (Luria Nebraska Neuropsychological Test Battery)
Weinberger et al. (1980)	51 schizophrenics	Lateral ventricular size (CT)	Poor premorbid function
Weinberger et al. (1980)	20 schizophrenics	Lateral ventricular size (CT)	Treatment resistance
Andreason et al. (1981)	52 schizophrenics; 47 controls	Lateral ventricular size (CT)	Negative symptoms
Takahishi et al. (1981)	169 schizophrenics 169 controls	Abnormalities of third ventricle, lateral ventricle, and cortex (CT)	Blunt affect, uncooperativeness

Note. CT = computed tomography.

in those with sulcal widening (Reider et al. 1979), and these groups were seen to be more impaired on many of the subscales (Donnelly et al. 1980; Lawson et al. in press). Several authors showed the Average Impairment Rating to be particularly higher (that is, show greater impairment) in large ventricle groups (Donnelly et al. 1980; Lawson et al. in press). The Mini-Mental Status exam, although not as sensitive an indicator of cognitive status as those previously mentioned, was also found by several investigators to relate to CT abnormalities (Nasrallah et al. 1982, 1983).

Most studies of CT abnormalities suggest that cerebral ventricular size in chronic patients is unimodally distributed and shifted upward compared with controls, and that patients with large ventricles may represent the extreme end of a continuum of pathology rather than a distinct subgroup. Crow and Mitchell (1975), on the other hand, suggested that patients who are disoriented to their age may form "a subgroup of severely incapacitated patients who, amongst other dysfunctions, have a defective capacity for acquiring new information" (p 362). Crow (1982) later expanded upon this theme to suggest two distinct forms of schizophrenia, type 1 having positive symptoms (such as hallucinations and delusions), no cognitive impairment, and normal CT scans; and type 2 having negative or defect symptoms (such as poverty of speech, flat affect, loss of drive), intellectual impairment, and CT abnormalities. Crow further suggested that the two syndromes proposed might have different etiologies.

It remains unclear, however, whether the constellation of signs and symptoms encompassed by the current diagnostic umbrella of schizophrenia reflects a dichotomous disorder, a continuum of pathology, or a more complex multidimensional illness. Nonetheless, consistent findings that structural brain abnormalities are indeed present in some patients and that these abnormalities are related to clinical manifestations (see Table 1) such as intellectual deficit, poor premorbid function, poor response to neuroleptic drugs, and negative or defect symptoms, strongly suggest that some schizophrenic patients suffer from an organic psychosis (that is, one having physical concomitants) of early onset and insidious progression to a deteriorated state, in other words, dementia praecox.

FUNCTIONAL BRAIN-IMAGING STUDIES

The data documenting abnormalities of brain structure in patients with schizophrenia and the relation of these differences to cognitive impairment have encouraged new studies of brain metabolism and physiology. These studies, aimed at delineating possible functional brain abnormalities, might elucidate the meaning of the structural abnormalities and clarify their relation to schizophrenic dementia. Studies of regional brain function (that is, physiologic, metabolic, and neurochemical processes) might also clarify where in the brain the dysfunction occurs in relation to the structural changes and how both relate to cognitive processes.

New methods for determining physiologic function directly in the living human brain have, indeed, yielded valuable and relevant data about schizophrenia. One functional imaging technique, the noninvasive Xenon^{133} inhalation method for measuring regional cerebral blood flow (rCBF), an indicator of neuronal metabolism and activity, has proved to be particularly well suited to investigating cognition in psychiatric disorders. The chemically and physiologically inert and freely diffusible radioisotope gas, Xenon^{133}, can be used as a tracer of rCBF, which in turn has been shown to be closely coupled with local metabolic rate and hence with neuronal activity. Xenon^{133} inhalation procedures are relatively quick, inexpensive, and easy to carry out and involve minimal radiation exposure. Therefore, a single subject can be studied a number of times under various cognitive or medication states to serve as his or her control.

Table 2 summarizes selected studies of brain physiology in schizophrenia that have been carried out using the Xenon^{133} inhalation technique as well as several other functional brain-imaging techniques. These include the invasive intracarotid Xenon^{133} technique developed by Ingvar et al. (1965) and positron emission tomography, which directly measures brain metabolism and chemistry. A survey of these studies reveals that consistent results have not always been obtained. In some cases, this may have been due to technical or conceptual limitations. Among the technical limitations is the use of methods such as intravenous or intraar-

Table 2. In Vivo Studies of Brain Physiology in Schizophrenia: Regional Cerebral Blood Flow

Study	Sample	Method	Results
Ingvar & Franzen (1974a, 1974b; Franzen & Ingvar 1975a, 1975b)	Up to 31 patients (all medicated), 15 controls	Intracarotid Xenon^{133} injection, resting and cognitive activation	Qualitative CBF distributional shifts (especially in older women): decreased frontal CBF, increased parietal CBF, no increased frontal CBF with activation
Matthew et al. (1982)	23 chronic patients (medicated), 18 controls	Xenon^{133} inhalation, resting	Decreased whole brain CBF (no P_{CO_2} correction); distributional differences
Ariel et al. (1983)	29 chronic patients (most medicated), 22 controls	Xenon^{133} inhalation, resting	Decreased whole brain CBF (no P_{CO_2} correction); suggested relatively decreased left frontal CBF
Gur et al. (1983)	15 patients (medicated), 25 controls	Xenon^{133} inhalation, resting and nonfrontal cognitive activation	No resting differences, laterality differences during activation
Gur et al. (1985)	19 patients (unmedicated), 19 controls	Xenon^{133} inhalation, resting and nonfrontal cognitive activation	Laterality differences during resting and activation
Mubrin et al. (1982)	17 patients (medicated), 18 controls	Xenon^{133} inhalation, resting	Decreased frontal flow only in elderly
Weinberger et al. (1986)	20 patients (unmedicated), 25 controls	Xenon^{133} inhalation, resting, regionally specific cognitive activation	Decreased flow to dorsolateral prefrontal cortex during specific cognitive demand
Berman et al. (1986)	24 patients (medicated), 18 patients (unmedicated), 17 controls	Xenon^{133} inhalation, regionally specific and nonspecific activation	Decreased flow to dorsolateral cortex only during specific activation; no medication effect

Note. CBF = cerebral blood flow.

terial administration and/or monitoring of the tracer, because these invasive procedures no doubt create cortical concomitants of their own that might obscure the intrinsic physiology being studied. Also technically limited are studies that have failed to take into account group differences in important variables such as arterial partial pressure of carbon dioxide (P_{CO_2}). Some researchers investigated only the so-called "resting state," which has been shown to be highly variable within as well as between subjects (Mazziotta et al. 1982; Wood 1980). Others have failed to control for medication or other state factors. Despite these limitations, a number of reports implicate dysfunction of the frontal lobe in schizophrenia.

One particularly sticky thorn in the sides of researchers investigating the frontal lobes has been a tendency to view this large brain region as a single homogeneous entity when, in fact, neuroanatomic and neurophysiologic studies have shown it to be heterogeneous (Fuster 1980). In our rCBF laboratory at the National Institute of Mental Health, we have designed studies to investigate the physiology of a particular part of the frontal lobes, the DLPFC (Berman et al. 1984; Berman et al. 1986; Weinberger et al. 1986). A variety of clinical and preclinical observations drew our interest to the investigation of DLPFC in schizophrenia. For example, this cortical region is not only uniquely developed in the human brain, but it is also the last cortical area to myelinate. It is even thought to continue to myelinate and to remain plastic throughout the entire adult life (Yakovlev and LeCours 1964). These considerations as well as numerous other factors, some of which are discussed later, render the study of DLPFC physiology especially cogent to the investigation of higher cortical function and make this area particularly intriguing to the investigation of schizophrenia.

Our approach to rCBF studies of DLPFC in schizophrenia is described here in brief. For each paradigm subjects underwent three rCBF determinations during three different cognitive states: The first procedure was always carried out during the resting state primarily to acclimatize the subjects; then, in counterbalanced sequence, the second and third procedures were carried out in conjunction with performance of the Wisconsin Card Sort, which was chosen as a DLPFC-selective task, and during performance of a simple numbers matching task designed to be exactly like the Wisconsin Card Sort in all aspects other than the abstract reasoning involved. The numbers matching task was administered under conditions identical to those of the card sort to control for the minimal finger movement necessary to make a response, the eye scanning and visual stimulation involved, and the subjective experience of taking a test while having rCBF measured. This strategy of serial testing of subjects and of tailoring a control task to those aspects of the rCBF landscape not integral to the DLPFC activity being studied allow the cortical metabolic concomitants of the DLPFC-selective card sort to be more specifically appreciated and quantified.

The resultant data (see Figure 1) indicate that normal subjects selectively activate DLPFC during performance of the Wisconsin Card Sort over the level of DLPFC activity during performance of the control task. In contrast, medication-free patients with chronic schizophrenia failed to activate DLPFC during the card sort and, in fact, tended to turn down DLPFC rCBF during the card sort compared with that during the numbers matching control task (Weinberger et al. 1986). The several autonomic measures of arousal that were determined during each rCBF procedure were not preferentially elevated for either task or in either group, suggesting that lack of arousal on the part of the patients cannot explain their DLPFC inactivity. Neither the Wisconsin Card Sort-specific DLPFC impairment in blood flow nor the patients' inability to carry out this task successfully were reversed by neuroleptic drug treatment (Berman et al. 1986). Furthermore, the degrees of DLPFC blood flow impairment and card sort cognitive disability correlated in the medication-free patients. Interestingly, patients made perseverative errors on the Wisconsin Card Sort, not random errors, and this inability to shift the conceptual set under conditions in which it is appropriate to do so has been classically described as a response mode characteristic of patients with DLPFC lesions (Milner 1964). In contrast to the Wisconsin Card Sort paradigm, during two versions of a visual continuous performance

Figure 1. Regional cerebral blood flow landscapes of left hemisphere mean grey matter blood flow for a group of medication-free patients with schizophrenia (bottom) and a group of normal controls (top) during performance of the Wisconsin Card Sort. Note the marked increase in blood flow (depicted as darker shades) in dorsolateral prefrontal cortex (DLPFC) (anterior pole at the left) for normal subjects. In contrast, patients show striking lack of DLPFC activity under the same conditions (from Weinberger et al. 1986. Used by permission.)

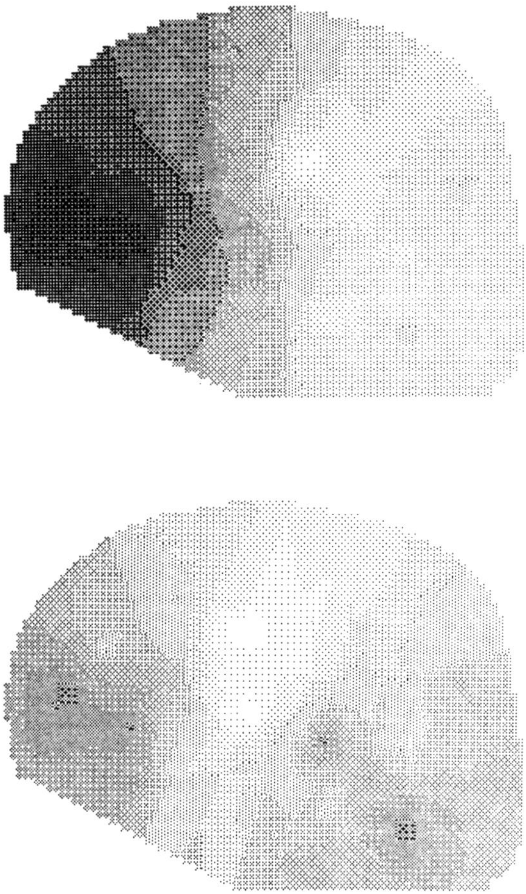

task, a test of selective attention not specifically linked to DLPFC on which patients with schizophrenia also do poorly, medication-free patients and controls were not found to have differing DLPFC rCBF (Berman et al. 1986).

Data from this controlled series of rCBF studies suggest that patients with chronic schizophrenia have impaired dorsolateral prefrontal cortical function that is specific to regionally selective cognitive processes. Furthermore, ventrical enlargement as seen on CT scan has been found to correlate with blood flow in patients with schizophrenia (Berman et al. 1985). This supports the notion that not only are subcortical structural and functional abnormalities associated with DLPFC linked but that they are also important organic concomitants of the dementia-like characteristics of schizophrenia.

PATHOPHYSIOLOGIC ASPECTS

The clinical, neuropsychologic, neurostructural, and neurophysiologic evidence reviewed provides insight into the nature of schizophrenic dementia. Interesting and potentially useful parallels between schizophrenia and other disorders with known pathology may be drawn and provide clues about where to search for central nervous system pathology in schizophrenia. For example, aphasias, apraxias, and agnosias, the hallmarks of most cortical dementias (that is, those in which there is prominent pathology in posterior cortical association areas) (Albert 1978) are not characteristic of schizophrenia. However, many aspects of schizophrenia are reminiscent of dementias accompanying frontal lobe disease or subcortical disorders. This observation recommends these areas for further attention in the study of schizophrenia.

Schizophrenia as a Frontal Lobe Syndrome

Patients with frontal lobe disease characteristically display many of the clinical signs and symptoms of schizophrenia. These include flat or inappropriate affect, lack of goal-oriented behavior, social dysfunction, poor insight and judgment, lack of concern for personal hygiene, minor (or "soft") neurologic signs, and disordered smooth-pursuit eye movements. The pattern of diffuse and usually subtle cognitive deficits noted in patients with schizophrenia is also quite similar to that seen in patients with frontal lobe lesions. Marked deficits in the ability to perform tasks such as the Wisconsin Card Sort are especially prominent in both patient groups. This deficit, as well as many of the aforementioned clinical features, are referrable particularly to the DLPFC.

The facts that cortical atrophy in schizophrenia may be most apparent in frontal cortex (Shelton et al. 1985) and that functional brain-imaging studies such as those described and summarized in Table 2 implicate altered frontal physiology in schizophrenia, support the idea of underlying frontal pathology in this illness. That physiologic and structural disorders of frontal cortex are correlated in patients with schizophrenia (Berman et al. 1985) is compelling evidence that these abnormalities are linked, and that they are important biological underpinnings of the disorder.

Studies of the development of DLPFC function, most of which have been carried out in nonhuman primates, have uncovered striking parallels with the development of schizophrenia; these may further substantiate the concept of DLPFC abnormality in schizophrenia. This area has been shown to be vital to the ability of postpubescent monkeys to perform delayed-response tasks, an animal equivalent of the Wisconsin Card Sort. Furthermore, electrophysiologic studies indicate that DLPFC neurons are specifically activated during the delay in the delayed-response task. However, DLPFC does not, at least in lower primates, come "on line" to subserve the performance of delayed-response tasks until after puberty (Goldman-Rakic et al. 1983). This is particularly intriguing in view of the well-documented peak in onset of schizophrenia in late adolescence. Perhaps many features of schizophrenia become clinically apparent only after DLPFC is called upon to carry out functions previously subserved by other brain areas. It is tempting to speculate that this feature of DLPFC development might explain the precocity (i.e., late adolescent onset) of dementia praecox.

Schizophrenia as a Subcortical Dementia

There are also striking similarities between the cognitive impairments in schizophrenia and those of so-called subcortical dementias. In 1974, Albert et al. coined the term *subcortical dementia* to describe the acquired intellectual deterioration of progressive supranuclear palsy, in which exclusively subcortical structures are affected. The syndrome is characterized by 1) forgetfulness (difficulty retrieving learned material), 2) mood or personality changes (apathy or outbursts of anger), 3) slowness of thought processes, and 4) deficits in manipulating acquired information (poor problem solving and impaired strategy and planning) (Albert 1978; Cummings and Benson 1984). Unlike most cortical dementias (for example, Alzheimer's disease), subcortical dementia does not include loss of basic language and calculating skills.

Although the concept of subcortical dementia is not without controversy, it has been extended to other neurologic illnesses such as Huntington's disease, Parkinson's disease, and other extrapyramidal disorders that involve primarily subcortical pathology and are accompanied by the relatively mild dementia described. The case for a role of subcortical structures in influencing neuropsychologic function has been supported by observations in animals and humans that lesions in specific subcortical structures produce identifiable cognitive deficits. However, attempts to use these observations to construct neuropsychologic test batteries that distinguish between cortical and subcortical dementias have been only marginally successful. Although patients with cortical pathology may score less than patients with subcortical disease on the currently used intelligence tests and mental status rating scales (Mayeux et al. 1983), both groups generally do poorly. Cummings and Benson (1984) suggested that current "tests used to assess cortical dementias are more well developed than those used to assess subcortical dementias. This reflects the fact that 'instrumental' functions mediated by the cortex (e.g. language, memory, perception) are more easily testable and measurable than the 'fundamental' functions mediated by subcortical structures (e.g. arousal, attention, motivation, mood)" (p 887). Thus, subcortical dementia, like schizophrenic dementia, has been difficult to characterize and quantify reliably (see Chapter 1 of this monograph).

A Dementia by Any Other Name . . .

Thus far, both frontal lobe and subcortical dementias have been likened to schizophrenic dementia. It is worth noting that frontal lobe syndromes and subcortical dementias are also strikingly similar to each other (Albert 1978). This is consistent with the fact that the neural circuitry of the frontal lobes may be unparalleled in degree of reciprocal connectivity with the limbic system and its subcortical correspondents (Nauta 1971). One implication of these dense reciprocal projects is that pathology of the frontal lobes will impact on subcortical areas and vice versa. Therefore, the substantial clinical overlap between frontal lobe syndrome and subcortical dementia is not surprising, and it would be incorrect to consider them mutually exclusive.

When viewed in this manner, aspects of schizophrenia suggestive of frontal lobe disorder and those implicating subcortical pathology provide a cohesive working definition for schizophrenia. It has been suggested (Weinberger 1984) that a more appropriate term for schizophrenia may be *frontolimbicopathy*. Regardless of the name used, it is clear that these brain areas and their intricate interrelations warrant considerable additional study in the investigation of schizophrenia.

FUTURE RESEARCH

Revolutions in biotechnology often precede new understandings in medical research. This has been the case in the application of techniques for in vivo assessment of brain structure and function to the study of schizophrenia. In the future, additional functional brain-imaging studies using methods such as rCBF, single photon emission computed tomography, and positron emission tomography, the latter of which can now quantify neuroreceptor function as well as local metabolic rate, will undoubtedly clarify the role of the frontal lobes and their subcortical correspondents in schizophrenia. Regarding new areas in the field of in vivo neuroanatomic study, magnetic resonance imaging has recently become available as a research tool. Magnetic resonance imaging, also referred to as nuclear magnetic resonance, is a technique for structural brain imaging that does not involve ionizing radiation and is capable of better spatial resolution and more versatile views of the living human brain than is CT. This technique has great potential to shed more insight on the concept of schizophrenic dementia.

The contribution of in vivo studies of brain structure and function to our understanding of schizophrenia can be optimized if combined with studies of cognitive function. For their part, neuropsychologic studies must be developed that better assess qualitative aspects of subtle disorders such as subcortical dementias,

Table 3. In Vivo Studies of Brain Physiology in Schizophrenia: PET

Study	Sample	Method	Results
Buchsbaum et al. (1982)	8 schizophrenics	^{18}fluorodeoxy glucose PET, resting	Slightly decreased relative frontal metabolism
Sheppard et al. (1983)	10 schizophrenics	O^{15}, CO_2^{15}, resting	No decreased frontal metabolism; laterality difference
Widen et al. (1984)	13 schizophrenics	^{11}C glucose PET, resting	Decreased parietal metabolism corrected with treatment, no hypofrontality, no laterality difference
Farchas et al. (1984)	13 schizophrenics	^{18}fluorodeoxy glucose PET, resting	Slight decrease in relative frontal metabolism
Buchsbaum et al. (1984)	16 schizophrenics, 11 affective disorder patients	^{18}fluorodeoxy glucose PET	Increased posterior metabolism trend to decreased frontal metabolism, no group differences

Note. PET = positron emission tomography.

frontal lobe syndromes, and schizophrenic dementia. These deficits can then be correlated with concomitant neuropathologic and neurophysiologic features in patients with schizophrenia.

REFERENCES

Albert ML: Subcortical dementia, in Alzheimer's Disease: Senile Dementia and Related Disorders. Edited by Katzman R, Terry RD, Bick KL. New York, Raven Press, 1978

Albert ML, Feldman RG, Willis AL: The "subcortical dementia" of progressive supranuclear palsy. J Neurol Neurosurg Psychiatry 37:121–130, 1974

American Psychiatric Association: Diagnostic and Statistical Manual of Mental Disorders (First Edition). Washington, DC, American Psychiatric Association, 1952

American Psychiatric Association: Diagnostic and Statistical Manual of Mental Disorders (Second Edition). Washington, DC, American Psychiatric Association, 1965

American Psychiatric Association: Diagnostic and Statistical Manual of Mental Disorders (Third Edition). Washington, DC, American Psychiatric Association, 1980

Andreasen NC, Olsen SA, Dennert JW, et al: Ventricular enlargement in schizophrenia: relationship to positive and negative symptoms. Am J Psychiatry 139:297–302, 1982

Ariel RN, Golden CJ, Berg RA: Regional cerebral blood flow in schizophrenia with the 133 Xenon inhalation method. Arch Gen Psychiatry 40:258–263, 1983

Berman KF, Shelton RC, Zec RF, et al: Frontal lobe structure and function in schizophrenia [New Research Abstract No. 1] 138th annual meeting of the American Psychiatric Association, Dallas, 1985

Berman KF, Weinberger DR, Morihisa JM, et al: Xenon^{133} inhalation regional cerebral blood flow: application to psychiatric research, in Brain Imaging in Psychiatry. Edited by Morihisa JM, Washington, DC, American Psychiatric Press, 1984

Berman KF, Zec RF, Weinberger DR: Physiological dysfunction of dorsolateral prefrontal cortex in schizophrenia: II. role of neuroleptic treatment, attention, and mental effort. Arch Gen Psychiatry 43:126–135, 1986

Bleuler E: Dementia praecox (The group of schizophrenics). Translated by Zinkin J. New York, International Universities Press, 1950

Buchsbaum MD, DeLisi LE, Holcomb HH: Anterposterior gradients in cerebral glucose use in schizophrenia and affective disorder. Arch Gen Psychiatry 41:1159–1166, 1984

Buchsbaum MS, Ingvar DH, Kessler R: Cerebral glucography with positron tomography. Arch Gen Psychiatry 39:251–259, 1982

Crow TJ: Two syndromes in schizophrenia. Trends in Neuroscience 5:351–354, 1982

Crow TJ, Mitchell WS: Subjective age in chronic schizophrenia: evidence for a subgroup of patients with defective learning capacity? Br J Psychiatry 126:360–363, 1975

Cummings JL, Benson DF: Subcortical dementia: review of an emerging concept. Arch Neurol 41:874–879, 1984

Dewan MJ, Pandurangi AK, Lee SH: Central morphology in chronic schizophrenic patients. Biol Psychiatry 118:1133–1140, 1983

DeWolfe AS, Barrel RP, Becker BC, et al: Intellectual deficit in chronic schizophrenia and brain damage. J Consult Clin Psychol 36:197–204, 1971

Donnelly EF, Weinberger DR, Waldman IN, et al: Cognitive impairment associated with morphological brain abnormalities in computerized tomography in chronic schizophrenic patients. J Nerv Ment Dis, 168:305–308, 1980

Famuyiwa O, Eccleston D, Donaldson AA, et al: Tardive dyskinesia and dementia. Br J Psychiatry, 139:500–504, 1979

Farchas T, Wolf AP, Jaeger J, et al: Regional brain glucose metabolism in chronic schizophrenia. Arch Gen Psychiatry 41:293–300, 1984

Feighner JP, Robins E, Guze SB, et al: Diagnostic criteria for use in psychiatric research. Arch Gen Psychiatry 26:57–63, 1972

Franzen G, Ingvar DH: Abnormal distribution of cerebral activity in chronic schizophrenia. J Psychiatr Res 12:199–214, 1975a

Franzen G, Ingvar DH: Absence of activation in frontal structures during psychological testing of chronic schizophrenics. J Neurol Neurosurg Psychiatry 38:1027–1032, 1975b

Fuster J: The Prefrontal Cortex. New York, Raven Press, 1980

Golden CJ, Gaber B, Coffman J, et al: Structural brain deficits in schizophrenia. Arch Gen Psychiatry 38:1014–1017, 1981

Golden CJ, Gaber B, Moses JA, et al: Differentiation of chronic schizophrenia with and without ventricular enlargement by the Luria-Nebraska Neuropsychological Battery. Int J Neurosci, 11:131–138, 1980

Golden CH, MacInnes WS, Ariel RN, et al: Cross-validation of the ability of the Luria-Nebraska Neuropsychiatric Battery to differentiate chronic schizophrenics with and without ventricular enlargement. J Consult Clin Psychol, 50:87–95, 1982

Golden CJ, Moses JA, Zelazowski R, et al: Cerebral ventricular size and neuropsychological impairment in young chronic schizophrenics. Arch Gen Psychiatry 37:619–623, 1980

Goldman-Rakic PS, Isseroff A, Schwartz ML, et al: The neurobiology of cognitive development, in Handbook of Child Psychology: Biology and Infancy Development. Edited by Mussen P. New York, Wiley, 1983

Goldstein G: Cognitive and perceptual differences between schizophrenics and organics. Schizophr Bull, 4:160–185, 1978

Goldstein, G, Halperin KM: Neuropsychological differences among subtypes of schizophrenia. J Abnorm Psychol 86:34–40, 1977

Gur RE, Gur RC, Skolnick BE, et al: Brain function in psychiatric disorders: III. Regional cerebral blood flow in unmedicated schizophrenics. Arch Gen Psychiatry 42:329–334, 1985

Gur RE, Skolnick BE, Gur RC, et al: Brain functions in psychiatric disorders: I. Regional cerebral blood flow in medicated schizophrenics. Arch Gen Psychiatry, 40:1250–1254, 1983

Haug JO: Pneumoencephalographic studies in mental disease. Acta Psychiatr Scand 38(Supplement 165):1–115, 1962

Haywood HC, Moelis I: Effects of symptom change on intellectual function in schizophrenia. J Abnorm Soc Psychol, 67:76–78, 1963

Heaton RK, Baade LE, Johnson KL: Neuropsychological test results associated with psychiatric disorders in adults. Psychol Bull 85:141–162, 1978

Holden JM, Forno G, Itil T, et al: Echoencephalographic patterns in chronic schizophrenia (relationship to therapy resistance). Biol Psychiatry 6:129–141, 1973

Ingvar DH, Congvist LR, Ekberg K, et al: Normal values of regional cerebral blood flow in man including flow and weight estimates of gray and white matter. Acta Neurol Scand 41 (Supplement 14):72–78, 1965

Ingvar DH, Franzen G: Abnormalities of cerebral blood flow distribution in patients with chronic schizophrenia. Acta Psychiatr Scand 50:425–462, 1974a

Ingvar DH, Franzen G: Distribution of cerebral activity in chronic schizophrenia. Lancet 2:1484-1486, 1974b

Jellinek EH: Cerebral atrophy and cognitive impairment in chronic schizophrenia. Lancet 2:1202–1203, 1976

Johnson EC, Crow TJ, Frith CD, et al: Cerebral ventricular size and cognitive impairment in chronic schizophrenia. Lancet 2:924–926, 1976

Johnstone EC, Crow TJ, Frith CD, et al: The dementia of dementia praecox. Acta Psychiatr Scand 57:305–324, 1978

Kaplan HI, Freedman AM, Sadock BJ: Comprehensive Textbook of Psychiatry III. Baltimore, William & Wilkins, 1980

Klonoff H, Fibiger GH, Hutton GH: Neuropsychological patterns in chronic schizophrenia. J Nerv Ment Dis 150:291–300, 1970

Kolb B, Whishaw JQ: Performance of schizophrenic patients on tests sensitive to left or right frontal, temporal, and parietal function in neurologic patients. J Nerv Ment Dis 171:435–443, 1983

Kraepelin E: Dementia Praecox and Paraphrenia. Translated by Barclay RM. Edinburgh, Livingstone, 1919

Kraepelin E: Textbook of Psychiatry [Sixth Edition]. Leipzig, Ambrosius Barth, 1896

Lawson WB, Waldman IN, Weinberger DR: Schizophrenic dementia: results of neuropsychological testing and clinical correlates. Am J Psychiatry (in press)

Levin S: Frontal lobe dysfunctions in schizophrenia: II. Impairments of psychological and brain functions. J Psychiatr Res 18:57–72, 1984

Lilliston L: Schizophrenic symptomatology as a function of probability of cerebral damage. J Abnorm Psychol 82:377–381, 1973

Luchins DJ, Weinberger DR, Wyatt RJ: Schizophrenia and cerebral asymmetry detected by computed tomography. Am J Psychiatry 139:753–757, 1982

Malec J: Neuropsychological assessment of schizophrenia versus brain damage: a review. J Nerve Ment Dis 166:507–516, 1978

Malmo HP: On frontal lobe functions: psychiatric patient controls. Cortex 10:231–237, 1974

Marsden CD: Cerebral atrophy and cognitive impairment in chronic schizophrenia. Lancet 2:1079, 1976

Mathew RJ, Duncan GC, Weiman ML, et al: Regional cerebral blood flow in schizophrenia. Arch Gen Psychiatry 39:1121–1124, 1982

Mayeux R, Stern Y, Rosen J, et al: Is "subcortical dementia" a recognizable clinical entity? Ann Neurol 14:278–283, 1983

Mazziotta JC, Phelps ME, Carson RE, et al: Tomographic mapping of human cerebral metabolism: sensory deprivation. Ann Neurol 12:435–444, 1982

Milner B: Effects of different brain lesions on card sorting. Arch Neurol 9:100–110, 1963

Milner B: Some effects of frontal lobectomy in man, in Frontal Granular Cortex and Behavior. Edited by Warren JM, Akert K. New York, McGraw-Hill, 1964

Milner B: Interhemispheric differences in the localization of psychological processes in man. Br Med Bull, 27:272–277, 1971

Milner B, Petrides M: Behavioral effects of frontal lobe lesions in man. Trends in Neuroscience 7:403–407, 1984

Mosher L: Schizophrenia: recent research trends, in Comprehensive Textbook of Psychiatry III. Edited by HJ Kaplan, AM Freedman, BJ Sadock. Baltimore, Williams and Wilkins, 1980

Mubrin Z, Krezevic S, Koretic D, et al: Regional cerebral blood flow patterns in schizophrenic patients. rCBF Bulletin 3:43–46, 1982

Nasrallah HA, Jacoby CG, McCalley-Whitters M, et al: Cerebral ventricular enlargement in subtypes of chronic schizophrenia. Arch Gen Psychiatry 39:774–777, 1982

Nasrallah HA, Kuperman G, Jacoby CG: Clinical correlates in sulcal widening in chronic schizophrenia. Psychiatry Res 10:237–242, 1983

Nauta WJH: The pattern of the frontal lobe: a reinterpretation. J Psychiatr Res 8:167–187, 1971

Owens DGC, Johnstone EC, Crow TJ, et al: Lateral ventricular size in schizophrenia: relationship to the disease process and its clinical manifestation. Psychol Med 15: pp 27–41, 1985

Reider RO, Donnelly EF, Herdt JR, et al: Sulcal prominence in young chronic schizophrenic patients: CT scan findings associated with impairment of neuropsychological tests. Psychiatry Res 1:1–9, 1979

Seidman LJ: Schizophrenia and brain dysfunction: an integration of recent neurodiagnostic findings. Psychol Bull 94:195–238, 1983

Shelton RC, Ingraham L, Weinberger DR: Cerebral structural pathology in schizophrenia: a new cohort. Abstracts of the Annual Meeting of the Society for Biological Psychiatry, Dallas, TX, 1985

Sheppard G, Gruzelier J, Manchanda R, et al: ^{15}O Positron emission tomography scanning in predominantly never treated acute schizophrenic patients. Lancet 2:1448–1452, 1983

Smith A: Mental deterioration in chronic schizophrenia. J Nerv Ment Dis 139:476–487, 1964

Takahashi R, Inabi Y, Inanga K, et al: CT scanning and the investigation of schizophrenia, in Biological Psychiatry. Edited by Jansson C, Perris C, and Strowe G. Amsterdam, Elsevier, North-Holland, 1981

Weinberger DR: Computed tomography (CT) findings in schizophrenia: speculation on the meaning of it all. J Psychiatr Res 18:477–490, 1984

Weinberger DR, Berman KF, Zec RF: Physiological dysfunction of dorsolateral prefrontal cortex in schizophrenia: I. Regional cerebral blood flow (rCBF) evidence. Arch Gen Psychiatry 43:114–124, 1986

Weinberger DR, Bigelow LB, Kleinman JE, et al: Cerebral ventricular enlargement in chronic schizophrenia: association with poor response to treatment. Arch Gen Psychiatry 37:11–14, 1980

Weinberger DR, Cannon-Spoor HE, Potkin SG, et al: Poor premorbid adjustment and CT scan abnormalities in chronic schizophrenia. Am J Psychiatry 137:1410–1413, 1980

Weinberger DR, Wagner RW, Wyatt RJ: Neuropathological studies of schizophrenia: a selective review. Schizophr Bull 9:193–212, 1983

Weinberger DR, Wyatt RJ: Cerebral ventricular size: a biological marker for subtyping chronic schizophrenia. Biological Markers in Psychiatry and Neurology. Edited by Usdin E, Hanin I. New York, Pergamon Press, 1982

Widen L, Blomgrist G, DePaulis T, et al: Studies of schizophrenia and positron CT. J Clin Neuropharmacol 7(Suppl):538–539, 1984

Williams AO, Reveley MA, Kolakowska T, et al: Schizophrenia with good and poor outcome: II. Cerebral ventricular size and its clinical significance. Br J Psychiatry 146:239–246, 1985

Wood F: Theoretical, methodological, and statistical implications of the inhalation rCBF technique for the study of brain-behavior relationships. Brain Lang 9:1–8, 1980

Yakovlev PI, Lecourse AR: The myelogenetic cycles of regional maturation of the brain, in Regional Development of the Brain in Early Life. Edited by Minkowski A. Oxford, England, Blackwell Scientific, 1964

Zec RF, Weinberger DR: The relationship between CT scan findings and neuropsychological performance in chronic schizophrenia, in Psychiatric Clinics of North America. Edited by Roy A. Saunders. Philadelphia, 1986

Zubin J: Chronic schizophrenia from the standpoint of vulnerability, in Perspectives in Schizophrenia Research. Edited by Baster C, Melnichuk T. New York, Raven Press, 1980

4

Depression and Dementia

Gerard Addonizio, M.D.
Charles A. Shamoian, M.D.

4

Depression and Dementia

Depression and dementia are disorders that share many common characteristics (Read et al. 1985). Clinically they may present in similar ways (O'Daniel et al. 1981). In addition, most severe depressions tend to peak in individuals between 40 and 65 years of age, a time when dementia begins to appear (Winstead and Mielke 1984). The prevalence of dementia in the elderly population 65 years and older varies markedly based on different survey findings (Gurland and Cross 1982). Rates vary from 0.5 percent to 31.8 percent (Gurland et al. 1980). In general, the rates for dementia increase with age; the greatest increases occur between ages 75 to 80 years. In one study, the prevalence rate of pervasive depression was 13 percent for people over the age of 65 years (Gurland et al. 1980). Both disorders have variable presentations and multiple causes, thereby creating even further diagnostic and conceptual confusion.

The term *dementia* refers to global cognitive disturbance, with no impairment in state of consciousness, which may be progressive or stable. *Reversible dementia* refers to potentially treatable conditions that cause intellectual deterioration but may revert to normal when the underlying pathologic process is alleviated. The causes of reversible dementia are extensive: intracranial conditions, systemic illnesses, vitamin deficiency states, endocrinopathies, drugs, heavy metals, toxins, infections, collagen-vascular disorders, and "functional" psychiatric disorders (Cummings et al. 1980; Roth 1978a; Small and Jarvik 1982). This type of disorder needs to be distinguished from the primary dementias. Multi-infarct dementia (MID) and Alzheimer's disease (AD) or primary degenerative dementia largely comprise this type of dementia, the latter being more common and both sometimes occurring concomitantly (Spar 1982). MID is caused by multiple cerebral infarcts, whereas AD is associated with marked pathologic changes: neurofibrillary changes, senile plaques, and granulovacuolar degeneration (Alexander and Geschwind 1984; Kosik and Growdon 1982; Plum 1979). Both disorders are progressive and result in intellectual decline, memory impairment, impaired judgment, personality changes, and disturbances in higher cortical functioning such as aphasia, apraxia, and agnosia. Depression may also be seen and is probably more common in MID (Post 1975; Rosen et al. 1980; Schneck et al. 1982). Except for brain biopsy or autopsy, there is no reliable diagnostic test for AD (Shore et al. 1983).

Not all memory disturbance in the elderly is secondary to pathologic dementing processes. Decline in memory function commonly occurs with normal aging. Kral coined the term *benign senescent forgetfulness* to describe this type of memory dysfunction (Kral 1962; LaRue 1982). "Malignant" forgetfulness, as seen in AD, is characterized by progressive memory impairment for recent experiences, a gradually increasing loss of remote memory, confabulation, and disorientation. In contrast, the benign form is associated with less overall impairment, minimal progression, variability over time, and an impaired recall of data associated with a previous experience without forgetting the event itself.

Depression is characterized by dysphoric mood, loss of interest or pleasure in usual activities, poor appetite, sleep disorder, psychomotor retardation or agitation, decreased sexual drive, loss of energy, feelings of worthlessness and guilt, difficulty thinking or concentrating, recurrent thoughts of death or suicide, and mood congruent delusions and hallucinations. As with dementia, depression may be associated with various medical problems (Dietch and Zetin 1983; Walker and Covington 1982). Depressed elderly persons frequently deny feeling depressed; rather, they may ruminate over somatic complaints (Gurland and Toner 1983). They may be so preoccupied with their ruminations that their concentration, memory, and thinking may become slowed and impaired (Gurland and Toner 1983). This impairment may become so severe that they develop depressive "pseudodementia," characterized by disorientation and gross memory disturbance and sufficient errors on formal psychological testing to overlap with scores of demented patients. Perhaps 15 percent of elderly patients with severe depression are seen with depressive pseudodementia (Gurland and Toner 1983), which may revert to normal with antidepressant treatment (Fann and Wheless 1981). Signs of cortical impairment such as aphasia, apraxia, and agnosia are usually not present (Cummings and Benson 1983). In addition to memory difficulties, there are many similarities between depression and dementia that can make the differential diagnosis quite difficult. Both states frequently exhibit apathy, anhedonia, social withdrawal, weight loss, anorexia, sleep disturbance, motoric slowing, and hopelessness (Miller 1980). In addition, errors in diagnosis may be based on diagnostic bias. A large international study of diagnostic differences in psychogeriatric patients demonstrated that New York psychiatrists tended to diagnose most elderly patients as demented as opposed to their colleagues in Toronto and London (Duckworth and Ross 1975). These differences stemmed from different diagnostic habits in the three countries. Nevertheless, the task of distinguishing between a severe depression and a moderate dementia may be formidable, especially when both disorders coexist within the same person.

HISTORICAL BACKGROUND

The relationship between dementia and depression is long standing and interesting. In the 9th century A.D. Rhazes, the Persian physician, cited melancholy as an inevitable condition in old and decrepit persons (Mahendra 1985). Later, dementia and pseudodementia received attention during the 19th century as reversibility, noncognitive symptomatology, and etiology were discussed

(Berrios 1985). Reversible dementia was explained by postulating the existence of "vesanic" dementia, dementia caused by functional psychosis. Meanwhile, Esquirol defined dementia as an acquired, irreversible, and severe form of intellectual dilapidation caused by organic brain disorder and chronic insanity (Berrios 1985). Mairet, a 19th century psychiatrist, coined the term ***melancholic dementia*** to describe patients with severe depression and cognitive impairment who frequently recovered despite the fact that Mairet thought their dementia was organically caused (Berrios 1985). He considered this condition to be a limited form of general paralysis. Descriptions of some of his patients suggest that they had depressive pseudodementia.

During the 20th century, the conceptualization of depression and dementia shifted. Dementia came to be considered an organic disorder, whereas depression was considered functional. We still struggle with this dichotomy despite the accumulating evidence of neurochemical abnormalities in depression. In 1952 Madden et al. (1952) coined the term ***pseudodementia*** to describe patients with disorientation and defects in recent memory, retention, calculation, and judgment that normalized upon alleviation of their psychotic condition. This pseudodementia was found in 10 percent of his 300 patients. None of these patients demonstrated witzelsucht, aphasia, or epileptiform seizures. Pseudodementia came to imply reversibility and functional psychiatric illness, whereas dementia implied irreversibility, progression, and degenerative brain disease. This concept of pseudodementia gained prominence with Kiloh's (1961) report of 10 patients. He felt that endogenous depression was the most common cause of an erroneous diagnosis of dementia, and that in most cases a sufficient explanation was a loss of concentration and inattention. Other causes of pseudodementia in his patients were the Ganser state, hysteria, malingering, paraphrenia, and mixed manic-depressive states. He noted that cases of pseudodementia, unlike dementia, have a short history and an abrupt onset. He cautioned against relying too heavily on pneumoencephalograms or psychological testing, and felt that clinical methods were still the most sensitive index in the differential diagnosis. The Ganser syndrome—one of approximate answers—was often discussed as a cause of pseudodementia, although this state may itself have various causes (Lishman 1978).

Wells (1979), noting that previous studies of pseudodementia based diagnosis on reversibility, attempted to define clinical features that might differentiate dementia from pseudodementia (see Table 1). He arrived at these factors based on a study of 10 patients ranging in age from 33 to 69 years. Wells noted that any one of these differentiating points was not diagnostically conclusive, and that the total clinical picture was the important factor. Although all of his patients performed poorly on one or more neuropsychological tests, inconsistent performance strongly argued against organic disease. Diagnostically, three patients had a typical depressive illness, whereas others had conversion reactions, posttraumatic neurosis, and schizophrenia. Pseudodementia may thus be associated with a variety of psychiatric disorders, not just depression. He noted that the most striking common feature of these patients was their marked dependency for physical care and emotional support. Importantly, pseudodementia was not reversible in all patients, thereby questioning the prior use of reversibility as a necessary criterion for the diagnosis.

Recently, the term pseudodementia has been critically examined. Folstein and McHugh (1978) considered it unsatisfactory for many reasons. They stated that pseudodementia patients are different from demented patients only in mood, not in cognitive aspects. In addition, pseudodementia patients share reversibility with many other types of dementia. Furthermore, considering these disorders as "pseudo" may hinder a search for potential biologic mechanisms. Folstein and McHugh pointed out that this syndrome is more common in the elderly and hypothesized that when a neurochemical disturbance of an affective disorder is superimposed on an old brain without a full complement of cortical neurons, this disturbance could provoke the cognitive disability. Folstein and McHugh suggested the term *dementia syndrome of depression*. McAllister (1983), in a similar vein, argued for viewing pseudodementia as a depression-induced organic mental disorder. Reifler (1982) also believed that the term

Table 1. Major Clinical Features Differentiating Pseudodementia From Dementia

Pseudodementia	Dementia
Clinical course and history	
Family always aware of dysfunction and its severity	Family often unaware of dysfunction and its severity
Onset can be dated with some precision	Onset can be dated only within broad limits
Symptoms of short duration before medical help is sought	Symptoms usually of long duration before medical help is sought
Rapid progression of symptoms after onset	Slow progression of symptoms throughout course
History of previous psychiatric dysfunction common	History of previous psychiatric dysfunction unusual
Complaints and clinical behavior	
Patients usually complain much of cognitive loss	Patients usually complain little of cognitive loss
Patients' complaints of cognitive dysfunction usually detailed	Patients' complaints of cognitive dysfunction usually vague
Patients emphasize disability	Patients conceal disability
Patients highlight failures	Patients delight in accomplishments, however trivial
Patients make little effort to perform even simple tasks	Patients struggle to perform tasks
Patients do not try to keep up	Patients rely on notes, calendars, and so on to keep up
Patients usually communicate strong sense of distress	Patients often appear unconcerned
Affective change often pervasive	Affect labile and shallow
Loss of social skills often early and prominent	Social skills often retained
Behavior often incongruent with severity of cognitive dysfunction	Behavior usually compatible with severity of cognitive dysfunction
Nocturnal accentuation of dysfunction uncommon	Nocturnal accentuation of dysfunction common
Clinical features related to memory, cognitive, and intellectual dysfunctions	
Attention and concentration often well preserved	Attention and concentration usually faulty
"Don't know" answers typical	Near-miss answers frequent
On tests of orientation, patients often give "don't know" answers	On tests of orientation, patients often mistake unusual for usual
Memory loss for recent and remote events usually equally severe	Memory loss for recent events usually more severe than for remote events
Memory gaps for specific periods or events common	Memory gaps for specific periods unusual[a]
Marked variability in performance on tasks of similar difficulty	Consistently poor performance on tasks of similar difficulty

[a]Except when due to delirium, trauma, seizures, and so on.
From Wells (1979). Reprinted with permission.

pseudodementia should be avoided. He stated that the term fosters a problematic organic-functional dichotomy when many patients have elements of both dementia and depression, and that it is often mistakenly used diagnostically. He feels that depression does not usually mimic dementia in a convincing way, and that the term *cognitive impairment* is more helpful than pseudodementia. Shraberg (1978) agreed that viewing dementia and depression as interrelated processes in the elderly is more useful clinically. It seems clear that we will continue to struggle with defining clinically more useful conceptual models until pathophysiologic mechanisms underlying the cognitive deficits of depression are understood.

Association of Dementia and Depression

A number of studies indicate how frequently patients diagnosed as demented receive a different diagnosis at follow-up. Marsden and Harrison (1972) studied 106 patients who were admitted with a presumptive diagnosis of dementia; of these, 8 were diagnosed as depressed, not demented. In 6 of the 8 patients, disturbance of memory was a presenting symptom. Kendell (1974) found a diagnostic change from dementia to depression in 8.2 percent of patients studied. Nott and Fleminger (1975) evaluated the course of 35 patients who had received the diagnosis of dementia upon admission to Guy's Hospital in London from 1950 to 1969. At follow-up, only 15 had deteriorated in a manner consistent with the original diagnosis. A significant degree of mood disturbance was found in both groups; a predominantly depressed mood was noted in 45 percent of the nondeteriorated patients. Ron et al. (1979) conducted a retrospective follow-up study of patients diagnosed as presenile dementia. Of 52 patients discharged from the hospital with this diagnosis, at follow-up the diagnosis was rejected in 31 percent. Ron et al. found that a previous history of affective illness and the presence of clear depressive mood at diagnosis was much more common in patients who did not continue to develop a dementing illness. Freemon (1976) studied 60 consecutive patients admitted for progressive intellectual deterioration and found that 18 patients had a treatable illness. Although many of these patients had a depressed mood, only 1 responded to tricyclic antidepressants with reversal of the dementia-like syndrome. Smith and Kiloh (1981) studied 200 patients admitted with the diagnosis of dementia. Ten patients were later diagnosed as having depressive pseudodementia, which had been present for two months to five years. They all responded to antidepressant treatment. Freemon and Rudd (1982) reviewed the records of 110 patients with progressive intellectual deterioration. Of these patients, 3 had a treatable depression. In an interesting study, Rabins et al. (1984) compared patients diagnosed as demented and depressed with those diagnosed as having irreversible dementia and those diagnosed as suffering from major depression. They found that a history of depression, report of depressed mood, self-blaming, hopeless and somatic delusions, appetite disturbance, and subacute onset identified the patients with dementia caused by depression. A two-year follow-up showed that coexisting cognitive impairment and major depression were not usual precursors to a progressive dementing illness. Alternatively, Reding et al. (1985) reported on 225 patients referred to a dementia clinic. Depression was found in 31 of 44 patients not considered demented, in 6 of 25 with some cognitive impairment, and in 24 of 156 with various forms of dementia. Follow-up of three years demonstrated that in 16 of 28 depressed, nondemented patients dementia later developed. Thirteen of these 16 patients had some sign of neurologic disease. Larson et al. (1984) prospectively studied dementia in 107 outpatients and found that patients with reversible dementia improved but rarely returned to normal. They argued that elderly patients with mental dysfunction are at high risk for various coexistent treatable conditions.

Further diagnostic confusion is created when dementia masquerades as depression, or "pseudodepression" (Feinberg and Goodman 1984; Morstyn et al. 1982). Kendell (1974) found that 23 of 870 patients originally diagnosed with depression later were diagnosed as demented. Sim and Sussman (1962) pointed out that depressive symptoms frequently appeared early in dementia, but these symptoms became obscured by the dementing process. This association has been confirmed by others (Gustafson and Hagberg

1975). Alternatively, Roth (1955) commented that an insignificant proportion of senile and arteriosclerotic psychosis begins with affective symptoms alone, and that the incidence of affective symptoms in senile psychosis is probably due to chance association.

All too frequently, dementia and depression are viewed in mutually exclusive diagnostic frameworks (Devanand and Nelson 1985). In fact, brief depressive mood swings are not uncommon in dementia (Kral 1983). Furthermore, major affective illness may occur concurrently with a dementing illness (McAllister and Price 1982; Reding et al. 1984). Liston (1977) examined records of 50 patients with a diagnosis of presenile dementia and found symptoms consistent with major affective disorder in one-half of the patients prior to final diagnosis. Depressive symptoms may be the earliest abnormality seen in dementia (Ziegler 1954) and may cause these patients to appear much more cognitively impaired than they would be without depressive symptoms (Ernst et al. 1977; Roth 1978b). In one study, Reifler et al. (1981) pointed out that when depression was ameliorated in patients with coexistent depression and dementia, cognition improved but there was a residual deficit. Rabins (1981) studied 16 patients with depression and found that these elderly patients were suffering from dementia as well. Reifler et al. (1982), evaluating patients in a geriatric outpatient program, diagnosed depression in 20 of 88 cognitively impaired patients. Seventeen had depression superimposed on an underlying dementia. Interestingly, the rate of coexisting depression decreased significantly with greater severity of cognitive impairment. Increasing age did not appear to increase the risk of depression associated with cognitive impairment. Reifler et al.'s data also argued against the view that depression is a common feature of early dementia, because two-thirds of the patients with mild dementia did not meet the criteria for depression.

Another important link between dementia and depression occurs in disorders associated with subcortical dementia such as Parkinson's disease and Huntington's disease. Depression and dementia are frequent complications in both disorders (Mayeux 1984). The clinical characteristics of subcortical dementia are psychomotor retardation, forgetfulness without inability to learn new material, apathy, and the absence of cortical signs such as aphasia or apraxia (Jeste et al. 1984). In contrast to cortical dementia as seen in Alzheimer's disease, there is improvement in psychomotor retardation, forgetfulness, and apathy, with support, reassurance, and encouragement (Jeste et al. 1984). Although the concept of subcortical dementia has been questioned (Mayeux et al. 1983), many investigators find it clinically useful. Some have likened the symptoms of pseudodementia to the type of dementing features seen in subcortical dementia (Caine 1981; Klerman and Davidson 1984). Caine (1981) reported that patients with pseudodementia frequently exhibit inattention, slowed mental processing, and a lack of verbal expression, which indicates an impairment of the cerebral structures that modulate higher cortical centers.

Focal brain lesions may cause not only cognitive deficits but disorders of mood and affect as well. There is evidence in humans that right-hemisphere function is dominant for many emotional functions (Bear 1983). In addition, it has been hypothesized that motor integration of propositional and affective language occurs in the brainstem while their higher integration occurs via callosal connections between Wernicke's area on the left hemisphere and its homologue on the right (Ross et al. 1981). Ross (1981) proposed that the affective components of language, including prosody and emotional gesturing, are a dominant function of the right hemisphere, and that their organization mirrors that of propositional language in the left hemisphere. Consequently, right-hemisphere damage results in various disorders of affective language, the "aprosodias" (Ross 1981). These lesions may distort the usual features of depression, including depressive affect, and make diagnosis difficult (Ross and Rush 1981). Ross and Rush (1981) proposed clues for diagnosing depression in neurologically impaired patients: poor or erratic recovery from neurologic insult; failure to cooperate in rehabilitation; clinical deterioration from a previously stable neurologic deficit; neurovegetative changes; pathologic laughing and crying in patients who do not have pseudobulbar palsy; and statements about dysphoria, guilt, hopelessness, and suicide even if affective behaviors are not congruent with statements. Robinson and Szetela (1981), studying 18 patients with left-hemisphere strokes, found that the severity of depression correlated with closeness of the lesion to the frontal pole, suggesting that depression may be a symptom of injury to certain pathways. Freeman et al. (1985) reported on a patient with depression, marked cognitive and behavioral impairment, and focal left-sided signs. All symptoms and signs resolved after electroconvulsive therapy. Clearly, focal brain lesions may dramatically change mood and affect; the precise pathophysiologic mechanisms remain to be elucidated.

Approaches to Differential Diagnosis of Depression and Dementia

Dexamethasone Suppression Test

Many studies in recent years have supported the hypothesis that early escape of plasma cortisol from suppression by dexamethasone differentiates endogenous depression or melancholia from other psychiatric illnesses (Raskind 1984). In one study of a large series of patients, the dexamethasone suppression test (DST) identified melancholic patients with a sensitivity of 67 percent and a specificity of 96 percent (Carroll et al. 1981). The utility of this test in diagnosing depression has been criticized, because weight loss alone in depression-free subjects may cause failure to suppress cortisol (Edelstein et al. 1983). A study by Reus (1982) indicated that DST nonsuppression is specific not to melancholia but rather to a subset of symptoms that may be present in different diagnostic categories. Nevertheless, a great deal of enthusiasm was generated over the possibility that we might finally have a biologic marker that would help in differentiating dementia from depression (Jenike 1983). The DST seemed to be helpful also in diagnosing post-stroke depression (Finklestein et al. 1982). It was found that advanced age did not appear to affect the DST in healthy humans (Tourigny-Rivard et al. 1981). Several case reports followed that indicated DST was useful in distinguishing pseudodementia from dementia (McAllister et al. 1982; Rudorfer and Clayton 1981, 1982). Grunhaus et al. (1983) found that combining the DST with the computed tomography (CT) scan was helpful in identifying pseudodementia. Several studies, however, have cast much doubt on the usefulness of the DST in differentiating depression from dementia. Raskind et al. (1982) studied 15 nondepressed patients with advanced AD and found that the DST was positive in 7 patients. Spar and Gerner (1982) found an abnormal DST in 9 of 17 elderly patients with dementia without depression. Coppen et al. (1983) demonstrated an abnormal DST in almost half of their dementia patients. Balldin et al. (1983) studied 21 patients with AD and 11 patients with MID. Twelve of the AD patients and 8 of the MID patients showed an abnormal lack of suppression. There was no correlation between depressive signs and postdexamethasone serum cortisol concentrations. McKeith (1984) found nonsuppression of plasma cortisol in 28 of 48 patients with AD and all patients with MID. These results could not be explained by associated depressive symptoms. Katona and Aldridge (1985), studying 20 demented patients, found failure of suppression in 10 patients. Interestingly, the nonsuppressive patients had a significantly higher score on a scale of signs of depression. In a similar vein, Carnes et al. (1983a) administered the DST to 33 elderly outpatients with the diagnosis of dementia. Fifteen of these patients would have met *Diagnostic and Statistical Manual of Mental Disorders (Third Edition)* (*DSM-III*) criteria (American Psychiatric Association 1980) for major depression if not for the presence of organic mental syndrome. Forty percent of these depressed, demented patients had abnormal DST results, whereas none of the 18 patients with dementia alone had abnormal DSTs. In another study, Carnes et al. (1983b) performed the DST on 26 elderly outpatients without depression. All patients had at least two medical diagnoses, and 14 were diagnosed as having dementia. No patient had an abnormal DST. The investigators noted that methodologic differences might have led to discrepant results from other studies. Their patients were outpatients and consequently may have suffered less stress, a potential cause of abnormal DSTs. Also, their patients were less demented than those of other studies. Jenike and Albert (1984) suggested that the DST is less likely to be positive in mildly demented patients. In their study of 18 nondepressed patients with AD, the DST was abnormal in only 1 of the mildly impaired patients but was positive in 4 of the 5 moderately impaired patients. These findings can be compared with work using the DST in post-stroke patients. In one study there was a significant correlation between total lesion volume and postdexamethasone 4:00 p.m. cortisol levels whether or not those patients with major depression were included in the analysis (Lipsey et al. 1985). Also, DST positive patients had significantly greater cognitive impairment than those with negative tests. Because there is evidence that brain norepinephrine is decreased in AD and depression, some investigators have suggested that this reduction leads to abnormal DSTs in both conditions by altering regulation of the corticotropin-releasing factor (Alexopoulos et al. 1985b).

Because the problem in differentiating dementia from depression is greatest in those who are mildly cognitively impaired, the DST may yet prove to be a useful diagnostic aid. Future research in this area needs to clarify this issue.

Electroencephalogram

Attempts at using the electroencephalogram (EEG) to differentiate depression from dementia have not been very helpful. Slowing of mean alpha frequency and the presence of a moderate amount of intermittent delta activity, particularly in temporal regions, has been regarded as part of normal aging (Harner 1975; Katz and Harner 1984). The onset of AD is usually not associated with marked EEG abnormalities, although there may be a slight slowing of alpha frequency or excess of delta activity (Harner 1975). With time, there is progressive diffuse slowing and a loss of fast activity (Alexander and Geschwind 1984). Nevertheless, correlation with the degree of dementia determined clinically is poor (O'Connor et al. 1979). There are also severely demented patients who have normal EEGs (Coblentz et al. 1973). The overlap between normal aging and dementia may be considerable. In one study of patients 60 to 79 years of age with either dementia or minimal symptoms, there was significant overlap in the mean alpha frequency although no patient with minimal symptoms had an alpha frequency that was lower than 8.5/sec (Harner 1975). In his classic work on pseudodementia, Kiloh (1961) mentioned that the EEG can be quite valuable in establishing a diagnosis, and that a normal EEG, especially with well-developed alpha rhythm, should suggest the possibility of a depressive illness. Ron et al. (1979) similarly found the EEG to be helpful in this differential diagnosis, yet Nott and Fleminger (1975) did not find the EEG helpful. In Wells's study, EEGs were recorded in 7 of his pseudodementia patients, and the results were normal in every patient (Wells 1979). O'Connor et al. (1979), studying patients with either AD, MID, or depression found significant group differences in power and coherence measures. Finally, although an abnormal EEG may not help distinguish between depression in the elderly and early dementia, a persistently normal EEG in a patient with continuing cognitive impairment should raise the possibility of severe depressive pseudodementia. Unfortunately, although there are significant group EEG differences in normal aging and progressive dementia, the diagnostic usefulness of the EEG for any particular individual is not great.

CT Scan and Pneumoencephalogram

Initial enthusiasm for the CT scan and pneumoencephalogram in differentiating between dementia and depressive pseudodementia has been dampened by significant overlaps in groups of patients. Dementia may occur without atrophy and atrophy without dementia (Kramer 1982). Similarly, normal elderly people may have enlarged ventricles, whereas demented patients may have normal ventricles (Jacoby 1981). Although a normal CT scan suggests a diagnosis other than AD, an abnormal scan may be helpful late in the illness when CT changes are quite obvious (Shore et al. 1983). Some studies have found a strong relationship between cortical atrophy and intellectual impairment (Ford and Winter 1981; Jacoby et al. 1980; Ron et al. 1979), whereas others have found that the size of the lateral ventricles predicts dementia more reliably (Ford and Winter 1981; Nott and Fleminger 1975).

Others have found clinical status to be a more reliable predictor of prognosis than CT findings (Ford and Winter 1981). Jacoby and Levy (1980a), studying groups of elderly patients who were either normal, demented, or had affective disorder, found that ventricular size correlated more closely with cognitive impairment in demented patients, whereas cortical atrophy was related to lower scores on a cognitive test in controls. In another study, the same authors identified a subgroup of affectively disordered patients with enlarged ventricles whose first depression began later in life and who showed more endogenous features (Jacoby and Levy 1980b). In a follow-up study, the researchers reported that these same patients had a significantly higher mortality rate (Jacoby et al. 1981). They also stated that this subgroup provides further evidence that organic cerebral factors may be important etiologically in some depressions of elderly people (Jacoby and Levy 1980b). In Wells's study of 10 patients with pseudodementia, of the 8 patients who had CT scans 7 were normal (Wells 1979).

More recently, attempts have been made to deal with the differential diagnostic problem between depression and dementia by assessing brain density through CT scans rather than making purely visual observations. Naeser et al. (1980) found this method extremely effective in distinguishing between groups of dementia and nondementia patients. Bondareff et al. (1981) found that mean CT numbers (Hounsfield units) were significantly lower bilaterally in the medial temporal lobe, anteriofrontal lobe, and head of the caudate in patients with dementia as compared with normal controls. Using a similar method, Jacoby et al. (1983) compared elderly depressed patients with healthy controls and patients with dementia. As a group the depressed patients resembled the dementia patients more than the controls, although there were differences among all three groups; controls showed the highest Hounsfield unit values, and demented patients showed the lowest. Yerby et al. (1985), measuring cerebral atrophy with digitized brain CT using a ratio of brain parenchyma to ventricular and subarachnoid space, found that this procedure's ability to differentiate persons with AD and those with pseudodementia was confounded by age. The authors concluded that this technique was of limited utility in resolving the diagnostic dilemma. Although the CT scan can be helpful in distinguishing groups of patients, for any particular individual its use in distinguishing between depression and dementia may not be very helpful.

Psychological Testing

Because cognitive impairment is frequently an integral part of the depressive syndrome, much work has been done to isolate those factors that may distinguish dementia from depression. Several studies have found general psychometric testing to be of little use in differentiating the two disorders (Kiloh 1961; Nott and Fleminger 1975; Smith and Kiloh 1981), whereas others have believed that certain types of cognitive impairment may be very helpful (Weingartner and Silberman 1982).

People with depression have various types of changes in cognition. Cognitive processes that have been demonstrated to be disrupted in the depressed state include attention, perception, speed of cognitive response, problem solving, memory, and learning (Weingartner et al. 1981). First, events in the past, present, and future are appreciated in qualitatively different ways. The depressed patient is usually preoccupied with past events and expects unfavorable events to occur. The depressed mood creates an informational context that determines how information is processed, encoded, and organized in memory (Weingartner and Silberman 1982). Events that were stored during a depressed state are less likely to be recovered under normal conditions, whereas those events that were stored under normal conditions are less accessible when depressed (Weingartner and Silberman 1982). Weingartner and associates reported that depressed patients used weak encoding strategies to organize and transform events to be remembered, thereby making the events less memorable (Weingartner et al. 1981). The investigators found that when the depressed patient was provided organization and structure, learning-memory deficits were no longer apparent. Furthermore, depressed patients have a general inability to sustain effort (Weingartner and Silberman 1982). Quantitative changes in memory also occur.

Strömgren (1977) studied memory in 152 patients with endogenous depression before the first ECT and after the sixth and last treatment. He found that endogenous depression impaired memory, and that recovery from depression eliminated the impairment. Others observed that there are differential hemispheric activation and performance effects associated with transient affective states (Allen 1982; Tucker et al. 1981). The Halstead-Reitan Neuropsychological Battery has shown evidence of right-hemisphere impairment in depressed populations with resolution of deficits with remission of depression (Weingartner and Silberman 1982). Kronfol et al. (1978) observed that depression interfered with cognitive functions largely subserved by the nondominant hemisphere, and that ECT delivered to either the right or left side improved those functions when the depression was ameliorated.

Some studies have shown that the severity of depression is directly related to long-term memory impairments, and others have shown a relationship with short-term memory (Weingartner and Silberman 1982). Sternberg and Jarvik (1976) found that depressed patients' short-term memory was markedly impaired but not long-term memory. The short-term memory improved along with the clinical state, but long-term memory was not influenced by therapeutic progress. One hypothesis is that depressed patients appear to have a memory deficit because they have a conservative response strategy, a low willingness to guess. Miller and Lewis (1977) examined this hypothesis by testing recognition memory function and found that when tested in this way depressed patients scored similar to controls, and both groups differed significantly from a demented group. In a similar vein, the "I don't know" response has frequently been used in distinguishing between depression and dementia, but recent research has demonstrated that such responses are also common in degenerative dementia (Young et al. 1985). In performing memory tests on depressed patients and others with altered brain function, Kahn et al. (1975) found that the complaint about memory was related to the level of depression, regardless of performance. Others noted that complaints about memory are a manifestation of depression rather than a reflection of a purely cognitive condition (Miller

1980). Depressed patients have great difficulty in memory and learning on tasks that lack internal structure (Weingartner and Silberman 1982). Although recall of random words differentiates depressed patients from the nondepressed, depressed patients, unlike those with dementia, are normal in their ability to learn inherently organized information such as semantically related words. Also, errors of omission are more evident than errors of commission in depressed patients (Cummings and Benson 1983).

Further complicating the problem of distinguishing between the cognitive deficits of depression and dementia is that both disorders may coexist. Breen et al. (1984), studying patients with either AD or AD and depression, found that depression did not worsen the short-term memory impairment associated with AD, although depression was associated with increased global intellectual impairment. Scales like the Hamilton Psychiatric Rating Scale for Depression are of questionable value when a patient also has dementia because demented patients have many neurovegetative features similar to depressed patients (Miller 1980). Although the Mini-Mental Status exam has been able to separate groups of patients with dementia and depression with cognitive impairment (Folstein et al. 1975), a new scale, the Cornell Scale of Depression in Dementia, has recently been developed to evaluate depression in people who have dementia (Alexopoulos et al. 1985a).

Although it is clear that depression is associated with many cognitive deficits, at this point there is no specific impairment that is pathognomonic for this illness (McAllister 1981). Psychological testing remains an important yet insufficient source of information in establishing a diagnosis.

Sleep Studies

It has been shown that age affects the length of sleep, its distribution, and sleep-wake architecture (Reynolds et al. 1983). In addition, rapid eye movement (REM) sleep latency decreases somewhat with age. Also, REM latency has been shown to be shorter in depressed patients than in patients with organic mental syndrome (Reynolds et al. 1980). Kupfer et al. (1981) found that in patients with endogenous depression treated with amitriptyline the application of EEG-monitored sleep criteria was more significant than clinical status in the prediction of clinical response. Other studies have shown that sleep EEG may be helpful in distinguishing patients with dementia versus depression. Two studies, one retrospective and one prospective, suggest that a shorter REM latency, greater early REM activity/density, altered temporal distribution of REM sleep, and greater sleep-maintenance difficulties are found in depressed, as compared with demented, patients (Reynolds et al. 1985a). Slow wave sleep may also be affected. Reynolds et al. (1985b) found that elderly depressives had a higher delta count per minute during the second non-rapid-eye-movement (NREM) sleep period than did controls or demented patients.

Other Approaches

Cerebral blood flow has been shown to be decreased in dementia (Hachinski et al. 1975) and in aging (Mathew et al. 1980). One recent study has examined cerebral blood flow in elderly patients suffering from either AD, MID, or depression (Hoyer et al. 1984). Patients with depression had significantly reduced average cerebral blood flow as compared with AD or MID patients.

Amobarbital interviewing has been used to distinguish between organic and functional impairments, because functional confusion purportedly clears with amobarbital. In anecdotal reports, it has occasionally been helpful in diagnosing pseudodementia (McAllister 1983). Alternatively, Cawley et al. (1973) administered barbiturates to depressed patients and found a sensitivity to sedating effects that reversed after therapy in proportion to the degree of clinical improvement.

Averaged cortical-evoked responses to auditory stimuli have been recorded in patients with dementia and depression. The latency of the auditory response was longer in demented patients than in controls, whereas depressed patients had intermediate latencies that did not normalize after recovery (Hendrickson et al. 1979).

Platelet monoamine oxidase (MAO) activity has been reported

to be increased in normal aging (Robinson and Nies 1980) and in AD (Alexopoulos et al. 1984b), but lowered in depressed women whose illness began at age 55 or earlier (Alexopoulos et al. 1984a). In a very interesting study, Alexopoulos et al. (1984a) found that patients with major depression and a reversible dementia had platelet MAO activity similar to that of depressed patients with AD. Both of these groups had higher platelet MAO activity than did patients with major depression without cognitive impairment. The authors suggested that a reversible dementia may develop when pathophysiologic changes associated with depression are added to an asymptomatic organic process associated with AD. Interestingly, Jenike (1985) reported 2 patients with AD and depression who failed to respond to standard antidepressants but improved with a monoamine oxidase inhibitor (MAOI). He suggested that high MAO activity in dementia may indicate that MAOIs have a special place in the treatment of depression in such patients.

RECOMMENDATIONS FOR CLINICAL EVALUATION

As stated in the preceding discussion, establishing a diagnosis in a patient who presents evidence of dementia and depression can be quite difficult. Both disorders may appear clinically identical, and they frequently coexist. Although group differences exist for clinical and biologic variables in patients with dementia and depression, using isolated diagnostic aids for any individual patient may create a false diagnostic impression. Using information from patient history data, physical exam, mental status exam, psychological testing, and laboratory procedures to develop a comprehensive picture will provide the highest probability of achieving an accurate diagnosis, although incorrect diagnoses may still be made. Long-term follow-up is critical, because resolving depressions and degenerative dementias will ultimately become manifest in a clearer way over time. (Also, see Chapter 1.)

Taking a thorough psychiatric and medical history from both patient and family is the first step. Previous history of affective illness and rapid progression of symptoms suggest a depressive disorder, although a gradual dementing process with a superimposed medical illness may cause an acute downhill course. Detailed information regarding medical illness, drug and alcohol abuse, and use of medicines must be clearly documented as these factors may be contributing to an organic mental syndrome with affective features. Similarly, a careful physical and neurologic exam may reveal a systemic illness that may be masquerading as degenerative dementia or depression. Signs of Parkinson's disease and stroke should be noted because both these disorders are associated with depression and cognitive decline. Laboratory screening includes complete blood count, sedimentation rate, blood urea nitrogen, glucose, electrolytes, vitamin B-12, folate, liver function tests, thyroid function tests, VDRL, urinalysis, electrocardiogram, and chest roentgenogram.

Several features of the mental status exam may provide clues to the differential diagnosis. Patients with depression, as opposed to patients with pure degenerative dementia, tend to exaggerate the extent of their memory problems, emphasize their disability, minimize their accomplishments, focus on past failures, consistently express depressive and somatic ideation, and make little effort to perform tasks. Depressive affect is frequently pervasive. Depressed patients may have a more erratic performance on memory testing than patients with degenerative dementia, and they are less likely to guess when they do not know the answer to a question. Psychological testing may be helpful, although there is no pathognomonic finding that will clearly differentiate the two disorders. Depressed patients are more likely to correct learning-memory deficits when organization and structure are provided and are more likely to do better on memory tests involving recognition. Also, evidence of aphasia, apraxia, or agnosia is frequently seen in patients with degenerative dementia or focal brain lesions but should not be found in a patient with a pure depressive disorder. The DST may be used but will be difficult to interpret because it is frequently positive in degenerative dementia as well as in depression. This test may be more helpful in distinguishing between mild dementia and depression because there is evidence that a lack of cortisol suppression with dexamethasone may be more common in advanced dementia. A normal EEG is helpful in ruling out toxic or metabolic processes. Also, a persistently normal EEG in a patient with continuing cognitive impairment should raise the possibility of a severe depressive pseudodementia.

The CT scan is extremely valuable in identifying structural lesions but may be less helpful in distinguishing between depression and degenerative dementia. Nevertheless, a normal CT scan with advanced cognitive decline should suggest depression as the source of the problem. When the evaluation is completed and diagnostic uncertainty remains, many patients will warrant a careful empirical trial of antidepressant medication. For patients with coexistent depression and degenerative dementia, such treatment may markedly ameliorate cognitive problems, although a residual deficit may remain. For all patients, long-term follow-up must be the mainstay of accurate diagnostic assessment and good clinical care.

FUTURE RESEARCH

If we are to clarify the relationship between depression and dementia, future research will have to be free of old conceptual frameworks. Continuing to think of the cognitive dysfunction of depression in terms of the old functional-organic dichotomy can only inhibit important associations between known organic illnesses and psychiatric disorders for which there is growing evidence of abnormal pathophysiologic mechanisms. Also, diagnostic certainty can no longer be based solely on reversibility because some organically caused dementias are reversible and some depressive disorders may be irreversible. The naive notion that someone is either depressed or demented will also have to be dispelled if diagnostic categories are to be accurately assessed.

A review of the past literature highlights the shortcomings of cross-sectional studies and the great need for long-term follow-up studies (Martin et al. 1983), not only to achieve more accurate diagnosis but also to assess the natural histories of these disorders. Completion of longitudinal studies of homogeneous groups of patients with autopsy and neuropathologic studies would allow important associations between brain anatomy, biochemistry, and clinical parameters. Rather than studying correlations of diagnosis to one variable, simultaneous assessment of imaging techniques, DST, EEG, sleep studies, psychological testing, and biochemical indexes would create the possibility of defining identifiable subtypes and achieving greater diagnostic certainty. It would also help to assess the clinical value of each of these tests.

Studies evaluating affect and mood in patients with focal brain lesions and subcortical dementia may lead to a common pathology underlying these disorders and the dementia of depression. A prospective natural history study of depression with cognitive dysfunction might clarify whether this disorder predisposes one to the development of AD or whether it uncovers a latent AD that has not yet become severe enough to be symptomatic. Correlating the natural history of these patients with those who develop depression without cognitive deficits could identify important subtypes of this illness. What types of treatment are most effective in depressive dementia and in coexistent dementia and depression remains to be elucidated. Certain somatic therapies may prove to be more appropriate and may provide clues to the underlying pathophysiology.

SUMMARY AND CONCLUSIONS

Based on the studies that have been reported here, it is abundantly clear that depression and dementia have many common clinical characteristics, in some cases appearing identical at any point. However, this is not different from so many other medical and psychiatric illnesses that present in similar ways. The danger is that our thinking may become encumbered by old concepts that reflect purely clinical phenomenology viewed in cross-section and neglect new sources of information that are becoming available with new technology. As we pay more attention to the course of illness and underlying pathophysiology, the current concepts of dementia and depression as we normally view them clinically may have to be revamped. There is nothing "pseudo" about the severe cognitive impairments of depression just as there is nothing "pseudo" about the affective disturbance in dementia. Such misconceptions can only prevent us from seeing possible relationships that could lead to greater understanding of the basic pathophysiology of both these disorders. The potential benefits of such an endeavor are enormous. The ultimate goal would be the development of treatments that could more specifically address what are probably a spectrum of disorders currently treated generically. Nevertheless, until this confusion is clarified, it is important to keep in mind that many of the patients who are relegated to the realm of "irreversible dementia" frequently have a treatable condition. The potential harm and suffering to patient and family of overlooking such conditions is all too obvious.

REFERENCES

Alexander MP, Geschwind N: Dementia in the elderly, in Clinical Neurology of Aging. Edited by Albert ML. New York, Oxford University Press, 1984

Alexopoulos GS, Lieberman KW, Young RC, et al: Platelet MAO activity and age at onset of depression in elderly depressed women. Am J Psychiatry 141:1276–1278, 1984a

Alexopoulos GS, Lieberman KW, Young RC: Platelet MAO activity in primary degenerative dementia. Am J Psychiatry 141:97–99, 1984b

Alexopoulos GS, Abrams RC, Young RC, et al: Cornell scale of depression in dementia [New Research Abstract No.124]. Presented at the annual meeting of the American Psychiatric Association, Dallas, May 1985a

Alexopoulos GS, Young RC, Haycox JA, et al: Biological studies in depression with reversible dementia, in Treatment of Affective Disorders in the Elderly. Edited by Shamoian CA. Washington, DC, American Psychiatric Press, 1985b

Allen RM: Pseudodementia and ECT. Biol Psychiatry 17:1435–1443, 1982

American Psychiatric Association. Diagnostic and Statistical Manual of Mental Disorders (Third Edition). Washington, DC, American Psychiatric Association, 1980

Balldin J, Gottfries CG, Karlsson I, et al: Dexamethasone suppression test and serum prolactin in dementia disorders. Br J Psychiatry 143:277–281, 1983

Bear DM: Hemispheric specialization and the neurology of emotion. Arch Neurol 40:195–202, 1983

Berrios GE: "Depressive pseudodementia" or "Melancholic dementia": a 19th century view. J Neurol Neurosurg Psychiatry 48:393–400, 1985

Bondareff W, Baldy R, Levy R: Quantitative computed tomography in senile dementia. Arch Gen Psychiatry 38:1365–1368, 1981

Breen AR, Larson EB, Reifler BV, et al: Cognitive performance and functional competence in coexisting dementia and depression. J Am Geriatr Soc 32:132–137, 1984

Caine ED: Pseudodementia—current concepts and future directions. Arch Gen Psychiatry 38:1359–1364, 1981

Carnes M, Smith JC, Kalin NH, et al: The dexamethasone suppression test in demented outpatients with and without depression. Psychiatry Res 9:337–344, 1983a

Carnes M, Smith JC, Kalin NH, et al: Effects of chronic medical illness and dementia on the dexamethasone suppression test. J Am Geriatr Soc 31:269–271, 1983b

Carroll BJ, Feinberg M, Greden JF, et al: A specific laboratory test for the diagnosis of melancholia: standardization, validation, and clinical utility. Arch Gen Psychiatry 38:15–22, 1981

Cawley RH, Post F, Whitehead A: Barbiturate tolerance and psychological functioning in elderly depressed patients. Psychol Med 3:39–52, 1973

Coblentz JM, Mattis S, Zingesser LH, et al: Presenile dementia—clinical aspects and evaluation of cerebrospinal fluid dynamics. Arch Neurol 29:299–308, 1973

Coppen A, Abou-Saleh M, Milln P, et al: Dexamethasone suppression test in depression and other psychiatric illness. Br J Psychiatry 142:498–504, 1983

Cummings J, Benson DF, LoVerme S Jr: Reversible dementia—illustrative cases, definition, and review. JAMA 243:2434–2439, 1980

Cummings JL, Benson DF: Dementia: a clinical approach. Boston, Butterworth, 1983

Devanand DP, Nelson JC: Concurrent depression and dementia: implications for diagnosis and treatment. J Clin Psychiatry 46:389–392, 1985

Dietch JT, Zetin M: Diagnosis of organic depressive disorders. Psychosomatics 24:971–979, 1983

Duckworth GS, Ross H: Diagnostic differences in psychogeriatric patients in Toronto, New York, and London, England. Can Med Assoc J 112:847–851, 1975

Edelstein CK, Roy-Byrne P, Fawzy FI, et al: Effects of weight loss on the dexamethasone suppression test. Am J Psychiatry 140:338–341, 1983

Ernst P, Badash D, Beran B, et al: Incidence of mental illness in the aged: unmasking the effects of a diagnosis of chronic brain syndrome. J Am Geriatr Soc 25:371–375, 1977

Fann WE, Wheless JC: Treatment and amelioration of psychopathologic affective states in the dementias of late life, in Aging (Volume 15). Edited by Miller NE, Cohen GD. New York, Raven Press, 1981

Feinberg T, Goodman B: Affective illness, dementia, and pseudodementia. J Clin Psychiatry 45:99–103, 1984

Finklestein S, Benowitz LI, Baldessarini RJ, et al: Mood, vegetative disturbance, and dexamethasone suppression test after stroke. Ann Neurol 12:463–468, 1982

Folstein MF, Folstein SE, McHugh PR: "Mini-Mental State"—a practical method for grading the cognitive state of patients for the clinician. J Psychiatr Res 12:189–198, 1975

Folstein MF, McHugh PR: Dementia syndrome of depression, in Aging (Vol 7). Edited by Katzman R, Terry RD. New York, Raven Press, 1978

Ford CV, Winter J: Computerized axial tomograms and dementia in elderly patients. J Gerontol 36:164–169, 1981

Freeman RL, Galaburda AM, Cabal RD, et al: The neurology of depression—cognitive and behavioral deficits with focal findings in depression and resolution after electroconvulsive therapy. Arch Neurol 42:289–291, 1985

Freemon FR: Evaluation of patients with progressive intellectual deterioration. Arch Neurol 33:658–659, 1976

Freemon FR, Rudd SM: Clinical features that predict potentially reversible progressive intellectual deterioration. J Am Geriatr Soc 30:449–453, 1982

Grunhaus L, Dilsaver S, Greden JF, et al: Depressive pseudodementia: a suggested diagnostic profile. Biol Psychiatry 18:215–225, 1983

Gurland BJ, Dean L, Cross P, et al: The epidemiology of depression and dementia in the elderly: the use of multiple indicators of these conditions, in Psychopathology in the Aged. Edited by Cole JO, Barrett JE. New York, Raven Press, 1980

Gurland BJ, Cross PS: Epidemiology of psychopathology in old age—some implications for clinical services, in The Psychiatric Clinics of North America. Edited by Jarvik LF, Small GW. Philadelphia, Saunders, 1982

Gurland BJ, Toner J: Differentiating dementia from nondementing conditions, in The Dementias. Edited by Mayeux R, Rosen WG. New York, Raven Press, 1983

Gustafson L, Hagberg B: Dementia with onset in the presenile period. Acta Psychiatr Scand (Supplement) 257:8–35, 1975

Hachinski VC, Iliff LD, Zilhka E, et al: Cerebral blood flow in dementia. Arch Neurol 32:632–637, 1975

Harner RN: EEG evaluation of the patient with dementia, in Psychiatric Aspects of Neurologic Disease. Edited by Benson DF, Blumer D. New York, Grune & Stratton, 1975

Hendrickson E, Levy R, Post F: Averaged evoked responses in relation to cognitive and affective state of elderly psychiatric patients. Br J Psychiatry 134:494–501, 1979

Hoyer S, Oesterreich K, Wagner O: Depression in old age and its relation to primary dementia: variations in brain blood flow and oxidative metabolism. Monogr Neural Sci 11:187–192, 1984

Jacoby RJ: Dementia, depression and the CT scan. Psychol Med 11:673–676, 1981

Jacoby RJ, Levy R: Computed tomography in the elderly: 2. Senile dementia: diagnosis and functional impairment. Br J Psychiatry 136:256–269, 1980a

Jacoby RJ, Levy R: Computed tomography in the elderly: 3. Affective disorder. Br J Psychiatry 136:270–275, 1980b

Jacoby RJ, Levy R, Dawson JM: Computed tomography in the elderly: 1. The normal population. Br J Psychiatry 136:249–255, 1980

Jacoby RJ, Levy R, Bird JM: Computed tomography and the outcome of affective disorder: a follow-up study of elderly patients. Br J Psychiatry 139:288–292, 1981

Jacoby RJ, Dolan RJ, Levy R, et al: Quantitative computed tomography in elderly depressed patients. Br J Psychiatry 143:124–127, 1983

Jenike MA: Dexamethasone suppression test as a clinical aid in elderly depressed patients. J Am Geriatr Soc 31:45–48, 1983

Jenike MA: Monoamine oxidase inhibitors as treatment for depressed patients with primary degenerative dementia (Alzheimer's Disease). Am J Psychiatry 142:763–764, 1985

Jenike MA, Albert MS: The dexamethasone suppression test in patients with presenile and senile dementia of the Alzheimer's type. J Am Geriatr Soc 32:441–445, 1984

Jeste DV, Karson CN, Wyatt RJ: Movement disorders and psychopathology, in Neuropsychiatric Movement Disorders. Edited by Jeste DV, Wyatt RJ. Washington, DC, American Psychiatric Press, 1984

Kahn RL, Zarit SH, Hilbert NM, et al: Memory complaint and impairment in the aged—the effect of depression and altered brain function. Arch Gen Psychiatry 32:1569–1573, 1975

Katona CLE, Aldridge CR: The dexamethasone suppression test and depressive signs in dementia. J Affective Disord 8:83–89, 1985

Katz RI, Harner RN: Electroencephalography in aging, in Clinical Neurology of Aging. Edited by Albert ML. New York, Oxford University Press, 1984

Kendell RE: The stability of psychiatric diagnoses. Br J Psychiatry 124:352–356, 1974

Kiloh LG: Pseudo-dementia. Acta Psychiatr Scand 37:336–351, 1961

Klerman GL, Davidson JM: Memory loss and affective disorders. Psychosomatics (Supplement) 25:29–32, 1984

Kosik KK, Growdon JH: Aging, memory loss, and dementia. Psychosomatics 23:745–751, 1982

Kral VA: Senescent forgetfulness: benign and malignant. Can Med Assoc J 86:257–260, 1962

Kral VA: The relationship between senile dementia (Alzheimer type) and depression. Can J Psychiatry 28:304–306, 1983

Kramer BA: Depressive pseudodementia. Compr Psychiatry 23:538–544, 1982

Kronfol Z, Hamsher K, Digre K, et al: Depression and hemispheric functions: changes associated with unilateral ECT. Br J Psychiatry 132:560–567, 1978

Kupfer DJ, Spiker DG, Coble PA, et al: Sleep and treatment prediction in endogenous depression. Am J Psychiatry 138:429–434, 1981

Larson EB, Reifler BV, Featherstone HJ, et al: Dementia in elderly outpatients: a prospective study. Ann Intern Med 100:417–423, 1984

LaRue A: Memory loss and aging: distinguishing dementia from benign senescent forgetfulness and depressive pseudodementia, in The Psychiatric Clinics of North America. Edited by Jarvik LF, Small GW. Philadelphia, Saunders, 1982

Lipsey JR, Robinson RG, Pearlson GD, et al: The dexamethasone suppression test and mood following stroke. Am J Psychiatry 142:318–323, 1985

Lishman WA: Organic Psychiatry—The Psychological Consequences of Cerebral Disorder. Oxford, Blackwell Scientific, 1978

Liston EH: Occult presenile dementia. J Nerv Ment Dis 164:263–267, 1977

Madden JJ, Luhan JA, Kaplan LA, et al: Nondementing psychoses in older persons. JAMA 150:1567–1570, 1952

Mahendra B: Depression and dementia: the multi-faceted relationship. Psychol Med 15:227–236, 1985

Marsden CD, Harrison MJG: Outcome of investigation of patients with presenile dementia. Br Med J 2:249–252, 1972

Martin BA, Thompson EG, Eastwood MR: The clinical investigation of dementia. Can J Psychiatry 28:282–286, 1983

Mathew RJ, Meyer JS, Francis DJ, et al: Cerebral blood flow in depression. Am J Psychiatry 137:1449–1450, 1980

Mayeux R: Behavioral manifestations of movement disorders—Parkinson's and Huntington's Disease, in Neurologic Clinics (Vol 2). Edited by Jankovic J. Philadelphia, Saunders, 1984

Mayeux R, Stern Y, Rosen J, et al: Is "subcortical dementia" a recognizable clinical entity? Ann Neurol 14:278–283, 1983

McAllister TW: Cognitive functioning in the affective disorders. Compr Psychiatry 22:572–586, 1981

McAllister TW: Overview: pseudodementia. Am J Psychiatry 140:528–533, 1983

McAllister TW, Ferrell RB, Price TRP, et al: The dexamethasone suppression test in two patients with severe depressive pseudodementia. Am J Psychiatry 139:479–481, 1982

McAllister TW, Price TRP: Severe depressive pseudodementia with and without dementia. Am J Psychiatry 139:626–629, 1982

McKeith IG: Clinical use of the DST in a psychogeriatric population. Br J Psychiatry 145:389–393, 1984

Miller E, Lewis P: Recognition memory in elderly patients with depression and dementia: a signal detection analysis. J Abnorm Psychol 86:84–86, 1977

Miller NE: The measurement of mood in senile brain disease: examiner ratings and self-reports, in Psychopathology in the Aged. Edited by Cole JO, Barrett JE. New York, Raven Press, 1980

Morstyn R, Hochanadel G, Kaplan E, et al: Depression vs. pseudodepression in dementia. J Clin Psychiatry 43:197–199, 1982

Naeser MA, Gebhardt L, Levine HL: Decreased computerized tomography numbers in patients with presenile dementia—detection in patients with otherwise normal scans. Arch Neurol 37:401–409, 1980

Nott PN, Fleminger JJ: Presenile dementia: the difficulties of early diagnosis. Acta Psychiatr Scand 51:210–217, 1975

O'Connor KP, Shaw JC, Ongley CO: The EEG and differential diagnosis in psychogeriatrics. Br J Psychiatry 135:156–162, 1979

O'Daniel R, Lippman S, Patel P: Depressive pseudodementia. Psychiatric Annals 11:43–50, 1981

Plum F: Dementia: an approaching epidemic. Nature 279:372–373, 1979

Post F: Dementia, depression, and pseudodementia, in Psychiatric Aspects of Neurologic Disease. Edited by Benson DF, Blumer D. New York, Grune & Stratton, 1975

Rabins PV: The prevalence of reversible dementia in a psychiatric hospital. Hosp Community Psychiatry 32:490–492, 1981

Rabins PV, Merchant A, Nestadt G: Criteria for diagnosing reversible dementia caused by depression: validation by 2-year follow-up. Br J Psychiatry 144:488–492, 1984

Raskind M: Biologic parameters in the differential diagnosis of dementia and depression, in Biology and Treatment of Dementia in the Elderly. Edited by Shamoian CA. Washington, DC, American Psychiatric Press, 1984

Raskind M, Peskind E, Rivard M, et al: Dexamethasone suppression test and cortisol circadian rhythm in primary degenerative dementia. Am J Psychiatry 139:1468–1471, 1982

Read SL, Small GW, Jarvik LF: Dementia syndrome, in Psychiatry Update, American Psychiatric Association Annual Review (Volume 4). Edited by Hales RE, Frances AJ. Washington, DC, American Psychiatric Press, 1985

Reding MJ, Haycox J, Blass J: Depression in patients referred to a dementia clinic—a three-year prospective study. Arch Neurol 42:894–896, 1985

Reding MJ, Haycox J, Wigforss K, et al: Follow-up of patients referred to a dementia service. J Am Geriatr Soc 32:265–268, 1984

Reifler BV: Arguments for abandoning the term pseudodementia. J Am Geriatr Soc 30:665–668, 1982

Reifler BV, Larson E, Cox G, et al: Treatment results at a multi-specialty clinic for the impaired elderly and their families. J Am Geriatr Soc 29:579–582, 1981

Reifler BV, Larson E, Hanley R: Coexistence of cognitive impairment and depression in geriatric outpatients. Am J Psychiatry 139:623–626, 1982

Reus VI: Pituitary-adrenal disinhibition as the independent variable in the assessment of behavioral symptoms. Biol Psychiatry 17:317–326, 1982

Reynolds CF III, Coble PA, Black RS, et al: Sleep disturbances in a series of elderly patients: polysomnographic findings. J Am Geriatr Soc 28:164–170, 1980

Reynolds CF III, Kupfer DJ, Taska LS, et al: EEG sleep in elderly depressed, demented, and healthy subjects. Biol Psychiatry 20:431–442, 1985a

Reynolds CF III, Kupfer DJ, Taska LS, et al: Slow wave sleep in elderly depressed, demented, and healthy subjects. Sleep 8:155–159, 1985b

Reynolds CF III, Spiker DG, Hanin I, et al: Electroencephalographic sleep, aging, and psychopathology: new data and state of the art. Biol Psychiatry 18:139–155, 1983

Robinson DS, Nies A: Demographic, biologic and other variables affecting monoamine oxidase activity. Schizophr Bull 6:298–307, 1980

Robinson RG, Szetela B: Mood change following left hemispheric brain injury. Ann Neurol 9:447–453, 1981

Ron MA, Toone BK, Garralda ME, et al: Diagnostic accuracy in presenile dementia. Br J Psychiatry 134:161–168, 1979

Rosen WG, Terry RD, Fuld PA, et al: Pathological verification of ischemic score in differentiation of dementias. Ann Neurol 7:486–488, 1980

Ross ED: The aprosodias: functional—anatomic organization of the affective components of language in the right hemisphere. Arch Neurol 38:561–569, 1981

Ross ED, Harney JH, deLacoste-Utamsing C, et al: How the brain integrates affective and propositional language into a unified behavioral function—hypothesis based on clinicoanatomic evidence. Arch Neurol 38:745–748, 1981

Ross ED, Rush AJ: Diagnosis and neuroanatomical correlates of depression in brain-damaged patients. Arch Gen Psychiatry 38:1344–1354, 1981

Roth M: The natural history of mental disorder in old age. Journal of Mental Science 101:281–301, 1955

Roth M: The management of dementia, in Psychiatric Clinics of North America, (Vol 1). Edited by Hendrie HC. Philadelphia, Saunders, 1978a

Roth M: Diagnosis of senile and related forms of dementia, in Alzheimer's Disease: Senile Dementia and Related Disorders. Edited by Katzman R, Terry RD. New York, Raven Press, 1978b

Rudorfer MV, Clayton PJ: Depression, dementia, and dexamethasone suppression. Am J Psychiatry 138:701, 1981

Rudorfer MV, Clayton PJ: Pseudodementia: use of the DST in diagnosis and treatment monitoring. Psychosomatics 23:429–431, 1982

Schneck MK, Reisberg B, Ferris SH: An overview of current concepts of Alzheimer's Disease. Am J Psychiatry 139:165–173, 1982

Shore D, Overman CA, Wyatt RJ: Improving accuracy in the diagnosis of Alzheimer's Disease. J Clin Psychiatry 44:207–212, 1983

Shraberg D: The myth of pseudodementia: depression and the aging brain. Am J Psychiatry 135:601–603, 1978

Sim M, Sussman I: Alzheimer's disease: its natural history and differential diagnosis. J Nerv Ment Dis 135:489–499, 1962

Small GW, Jarvik LF: The dementia syndrome. Lancet 2:1443–1446, 1982

Smith JS, Kiloh LG: The investigation of dementia: results in 200 consecutive admissions. Lancet 1:824–827, 1981

Spar JE: Dementia in the aged, in Psychiatric Clinics of North America (Vol 5). Edited by Jarvik LF, Small GW. Philadelphia, Saunders, 1982

Spar JE, Gerner R: Does the dexamethasone suppression test distinguish dementia from depression? Am J Psychiatry 139:238–240, 1982

Sternberg DE, Jarvik ME: Memory function in depression-improvement with antidepressant medication. Arch Gen Psychiatry 33:219–224, 1976

Stromgren LS: The influence of depression on memory. Acta Psychiatr Scand 56:109–128, 1977

Tourigny-Rivard M, Raskind M, Rivard D: The dexamethasone suppression test in an elderly population. Biol Psychiatry 16:1177–1184, 1981

Tucker DM, Stenslie CE, Roth RS, et al: Right frontal lobe activation and right hemisphere performance—decrement during a depressed mood. Arch Gen Psychiatry 38:169–174, 1981

Walker JI, Covington TR: Therapy review: diagnosis and pharmacological management of depression in the elderly. Journal of Clinical and Experimental Gerontology 4:1–39, 1982

Weingartner H, Cohen RM, Murphy DL, et al: Cognitive processes in depression. Arch Gen Psychiatry 38:42–47, 1981

Weingartner H, Silberman E: Models of cognitive impairment: cognitive changes in depression. Psychopharmacol Bull 18:27–42, 1982

Wells CE: Pseudodementia. Am J Psychiatry 136:895–900, 1979

Winstead DK, Mielke DH: Differential diagnosis between dementia and depression in the elderly, in Neurologic Clinics (Volume 2). Edited by Green JB. Philadelphia, Saunders, 1984

Yerby MS, Sundsten JW, Larson EB, et al: A new method of measuring brain atrophy: the effect of aging in its application for diagnosing dementia. Neurology 35:1316–1320, 1985

Young, RC, Manley MW, Alexopoulos GS: "I don't know" responses in elderly depressives and in dementia. J Am Geriatr Soc 33:253–257, 1985

Ziegler DK: Cerebral atrophy in psychiatric patients. Am J Psychiatry 111:454–458, 1954

5

Neuronal Loss in Normal Aging and Neuropsychiatric Dementias

Dilip V. Jeste, M.D.
James B. Lohr, M.D.
Ranjit B. Mani, M.D.
Jean Lud Cadet, M.D.
Carol Ludwig, M.D.

5

Neuronal Loss in Normal Aging and Neuropsychiatric Dementias

Simple as well as complex behavior reflects brain function. Kandel (1981) reviewed the history of the dispute between two alternate views on the relationship between brain and behavior. One theory —the aggregate field view—argues that various higher functions are not localized to specific regions in the cerebral cortex; rather, the cortex acts as a whole for each of its mental functions. Accordingly, lesions of any part of the cortex would affect all the higher functions equally. The competing hypothesis, which is now widely accepted, is called the theory of cellular connectionism. It states that specific behaviors are mediated by specific brain regions through localized pathways, so that lesions of different brain regions would produce different behavioral effects. Around the turn of this century, Cajal proposed that the histologic basis of behavior could be explained with the neuron doctrine, according to which the structural and functional unit of the nervous system was a neuron (see Kandel 1981).

Three authors (Drs. Jeste, Lohr, and Cadet) contributed to this chapter in their personal capacity. This chapter, therefore, does not necessarily reflect the views of the National Institute of Mental Health.

We wish to thank Mohamad Haleem, Curator of the Yakovlev Collection, and members of the staff of the Department of Neuropathology at the Armed Forces Institute of Pathology, Washington, D.C., for their help in the neuronometric studies performed there.

The hypothesis of cellular connections and the neuron doctrine provide the rationale for seeking associations between specific behavioral deficits and neuronal lesions in given parts of the brain. The final stage of neuronal damage is the disappearance of a neuron. Furthermore, neuronal loss in individual brain areas lends itself to objective and quantifiable measurements. We should stress at the outset, however, that lesions not producing neuronal drop-out could still cause neuronal dysfunction (for example, disturbances of neurotransmitter activities). Hence, neuronal loss should be viewed as only one of the major components of neuropathology of specific brain disorders.

A number of investigators reported various neuropathologic changes in normal aging, Alzheimer's disease, Parkinson's disease, Huntington's disease, schizophrenia, and other conditions that may be associated with dementia. One common although not always consistent finding in all these conditions is that of neuronal loss in specific, albeit different, areas of the brain. This chapter focuses on studies of neuronal dropout in normal aging and in certain dementing disorders. First, we present a general introduction to the field of quantitative neuronometry and aging. Second, we review the literature on quantitative studies of neuronal loss in normal human aging. Then we discuss some of our own recent work on the quantitative neuropathology of normal aging in the cerebellum and hippocampus. Fourth, we discuss an hypothesis on the pathophysiology of neuron loss in aging. Finally, we offer a brief overview of neuronal loss in certain neuropsychiatric dementias.

QUANTITATIVE NEURONOMETRY AND AGING

There is a general impression in the scientific community that as the brain ages neurons die. This idea first received experimental support in the late 1800s with Hodge's (1894) neuronometric studies on honeybee brains. Hodge discovered that the ratio of the number of neurons in young versus old brains was nearly 3:1, suggesting that as many as two-thirds of the neurons in these insect brains had disappeared over their lifetime. Despite the fact that a number of subsequent studies failed to support the idea of aging-related neuron loss (Konigsmark and Murphy 1970; Monagle and Brody 1974; Van Buskirk 1945; Vijayashankar and Brody 1977), the notion continues to have widespread acceptance and appeal. Many scientists still quote the Burns (1958) statement that every day of our adult lives as many as 100,000 neurons die, even though this statement was based on a comparison of two unrelated studies (Brody 1955; Leboucq 1929), neither of which made such a claim (Brody 1978).

Recently, the idea that aging is inevitably associated with neuron loss has been formally challenged (see Kemper 1984). Comfort (1971) referred to the concept of aging-related neuronal loss as possibly being nothing more than "neuromythology." Overall, it appears that such neuron loss varies greatly from one region of the brain to another. Some areas of the brain may not lose neurons at all. In the granular layer of the rat hippocampus, there is evidence that neurons may actually *increase* in number with age (Bayer et al. 1982).

In Table 1 is presented a list of studies that have attempted to determine quantitatively changes in neuronal count or density with age in the human brain. The total number of studies is surprisingly small considering the large number of different brain regions, and there are rarely more than two or three studies on any given brain region, which makes interpretation difficult.

Additional problems in analyzing quantitative studies pertain to methodology, which has varied considerably from study to study. This may be due in part to the vast number of neurons in the brain (probably in the trillions), which forces investigators to measure relatively small representative regions and to assume that their results hold true for larger areas. These procedures are most accurate for small brain regions such as brainstem nuclei, where the whole structure can be sectioned and a large percentage of the total number of neurons can be counted.

There are also different approaches to counting neurons in the brain. One, used by many researchers, involves selecting a small representative sample region from a much larger area and counting the number of cells on a slide from that region. The results are then expressed in cells per unit area (for example, cells/mm^2). Some researchers take their investigations one step further by measuring a third dimension (often the depth of the tissue) to express their results as cells per unit volume (for example, cells/mm^3). If the total volume of the brain region is known, an approximation of the total number of neurons may be made, assuming that the neuronal density remains constant throughout the region. One of the problems with quantitative measurements of neuronal density in a given area (without estimating volume) is that any change in volume of that area with age will affect the relationship of age and neuron density whether or not there is an actual neuron loss. In most brain regions, the volume probably decreases with age (see Hall et al. 1975; Haug et al. 1983; Hopker 1951), but in some regions an increase may occur such as that described by Konigsmark and Murphy (1972) in the ventral cochlear nucleus. Therefore, an increase or decrease in neuron density may reflect tissue shrinkage or expansion and not necessarily changes in the total number of neurons.

Some investigators have measured the number of neurons per gram of tissue by ultrasonically disrupting brain tissue and separating the neurons from other cells using centrifugation. This procedure was used in the studies of Devaney and Johnson (1980, 1984). The advantage of the technique is that small intraregional variations in neuron density are automatically averaged. It shares, however, several problems with other measurement procedures, and in addition, it is difficult to identify cell types following tissue disruption and centrifugation.

Despite some limitations, quantitative neuronometric techniques, because they are less susceptible to the problems associated with subjective assessment of neuronal density, offer an advantage over qualitative methods. This is illustrated in Figure 1. The densities of dots in square A and square B are different, but it is difficult to state the exact difference by a mere subjective estimation of their densities. In actuality, the areal density of A is 25 percent less than that of B, although qualitative examiners have given estimates ranging from no difference to a 50 percent difference in density. If A and B were not juxtaposed, it would be even

Table 1. Aging-Related Neuronal Loss in Various Areas of the Human Brain

Region	Measurement	Number of subjects	Age range (years)	% loss of neurons over age range	% loss of neurons from age 20 to 100[a]	Study
CEREBRAL CORTEX						
Frontal lobe						
Area 10 (prefrontal)	Total neuron number (layer III)	15	19 to >77[b]	28.0	44.8	Shefer (1972)
Area 10 (prefrontal)	Number of neurons/ unit volume	4	Adolescence to 85	44.0	50.4	Colon (1972)
Area 11 (orbitofrontal)	Total neuron number	40	21 to 111	30.6	27.2	Haug et al. (1983)
Area 9 (superior frontal gyrus)	Number of neurons/full thickness slab of cortex[c]	18	41 to 87	35.6	62.4	Brody (1970)
Area 6 (premotor)	Total neuron number (layer III)	15	19 to >77[b]	22.0	35.2	Shefer (1972)
Area 6 (premotor)	Total neuron number[d]	40	21 to 111	0.9	0.8	Haug et al. (1983)
Area 4 (precentral gyrus)	Number of neurons/ full thickness	16	16 to 95[e]	38.3	38.4	Brody (1955)
Area 4 (precentral gyrus)	Number of neurons/ unit volume	4	Adolescence to 85	44.0	50.4	Colon (1972)
Area 4 (precentral gyrus)	Number of neurons/unit area (small and large neurons)	66	18 to 95	48.0	49.9	Henderson et al. (1980)
Temporal lobe						
Area 22 (superior temporal gyrus)	Number of neurons/ full thickness	16	16 to 95[e]	57.5	57.6	Brody (1955)

Area 22 (superior temporal gyrus)	Number of neurons/unit area (small and large neurons)	66	18 to 95	47.2	49.1	Henderson et al. (1980)
Area 21 (middle temporal gyrus)	Total neuron number (layer III)	15	19 to >77[b]	23.0	36.8	Shefer (1972)
Area 21/38	Total neuron number (layer III)	15	19 to >77[b]	12.0	19.2	Shefer (1972)
Area 20	Number of neurons/unit area (small and large neurons)	66	18 to 95	26.4	27.4	Henderson et al. (1980)
Parietal lobe						
Areas 3,1,2 (postcentral gyrus)	Number of neurons/full thickness slab of cortex[c]	16	16 to 95[e]	0.0	0.0	Brody (1955)
Areas 3,1,2 (postcentral gyrus)	Number of neurons/unit area (small and large neurons)	66	18 to 95	51.7	53.7	Henderson et al. (1980)
Area 40	Total neuron number (layer III)	15	19 to >77[b]	15.0	24.0	Shefer (1972)
Area 7	Total neuron number[d]	40	21 to 111	0.0	0.0	Haug et al. (1983)
Occipital lobe						
Area 18	Total neuron number (layer III)	15	19 to >77[b]	13.5	21.6	Shefer (1972)
Area 17	Number of neurons/full thickness slab of cortex[c]	16	16 to 95[e]	39.1	39.2	Brody (1955)
Area 17	Number of neurons/ unit volume	4	Adolescence to 85	44.0	50.4	Colon (1972)
Area 17	Total neuron number[d]	40	21 to 111	0.0[f]	0.0[f]	Haug et al. (1983)
Macular area	Number of neurons/g	23	20 to 87	46.2	55.2	Devaney and Johnson (1980)

Table 1. Aging-Related Neuronal Loss in Various Areas of the Human Brain *(continued)*

Region	Measurement	Number of subjects	Age range (years)	% loss of neurons over age range	% loss of neurons from age 20 to 100[a]	Study
Other areas						
Area 24 (cingulate gyrus)	Number of neurons/ unit volume	4	Adolescence to 85	44.0	50.4	Colon (1972)
Area 28 (subiculum)	Total neuron number	15	19 to >77[b]	29.0	46.4	Shefer (1977)
Gyrus rectus	Number of neurons/unit area (small and large neurons)	66	18 to 95	40.1	41.7	Henderson et al. (1980)
SUBCORTICAL REGIONS						
Amygdala (lateral and superficial cortical nuclei)	Number of neurons/mm^3	8	20 to 76	16.2	23.2	Herzog and Kemper (1980)
Medical nuclei	Number of neurons/mm^3	8	20 to 76	40.9	58.4	Herzog and Kemper (1980)
Medical portion of central nucleus	Number of neurons/mm^3	8	20 to 76	27.4	39.2	Herzog and Kemper (1980)
All other nuclei	Number of neurons/mm^3	8	20 to 76	0.0	0.0	Herzog and Kemper (1980)
Hippocampus	Number of pyramidal neurons/ mm^3	18	47 to 91	23.8	43.2	Ball (1977)
Hippocampus	Number of pyramidal neurons/ mm^3	40	21 to 91	34.2	39.0	Dam (1979)
Hippocampus	Number of neurons/g	25	20 to 87	0.0[f]	0.0[f]	Devaney and Johnson (1984)

Hippocampus	Number of pyramidal cells/mm^2	23	4 to 98	36.0 (in CA4)	30.4 (in CA4)	Mani et al. (in press)
Mammillary bodies	Total neuron number	15	27 to 84	0.0	0.0	Wilkinson and Davies (1978)
Nucleus basalis	Neuronal counts	9	44 to 78	0.0	0.0	Rogers et al. (1985)
Nucleus basalis	Total neuron number	30	40 to 88	0.0	0.0	Whitehouse et al. (1983b)
Basal forebrain cholinergic cells	Total neuron number	11	Up to 95	57.0	60.0	McGeer et al. (1984a)
Putamen	Number of large neurons/mm^3	14	Newborn to 65	35.8	44.0	Bugiani et al. (1978)
	Number of small neurons/mm^3	14	Newborn to 65	54.0	66.4	Bugiani et al. (1978)
CEREBELLUM						
Cerebellar hemispheres	Number of Purkinje cells/unit volume (corrected to be an index of total number of Purkinje cells)	5	42 to 100	37.1	51.2	Ellis (1919)
Cerebellar hemispheres	Number of Purkinje cells/unit volume (corrected to be an index of total number of Purkinje cells)	10	19 to 92	30.7	33.6	Ellis (1920)

Table 1. Aging-Related Neuronal Loss in Various Areas of the Human Brain *(continued)*

Region	Measurement	Number of subjects	Age range (years)	% loss of neurons over age range	% loss of neurons from age 20 to 100[a]	Study
Cerebellar hemispheres	Not stated	6	6 to 85	0.0	0.0	Delorenzi (1931)
Cerebellar hemispheres	Proportion of total population (a value related to total number of Purkinje cells)	90	Newborn to 110	27.7	20.1	Hall et al. (1975)
Cerebellar hemispheres	Number of Purkinje cells/mm	47	3 to 98	46.6	39.2	Jeste et al. (in press)
Anterior vermis	Number of Purkinje cells/ mm of folium	46	3 to 98	54.2	45.6	Jeste et al. (in press)
Posterior vermis	Number of Purkinje cells/ mm of folium	46	3 to 98	50.4	42.4	Jeste et al. (in press)
Dentate nucleus	Number of large neurons	27	6 to 99	0.0	0.0	Hopker (1951)
Dentate nucleus	Number of cells	3	30 months to 45 years	0.0	0.0	Heidary and Tomasch (1969)
Dentate nucleus	Number of multipolar cells/mm^2	46	3 to 98	0.0	0.0	Jeste et al. (in press)
BRAINSTEM						
Substantia nigra	Total neuron number	13	5 to 90	57.8	54.4	McGeer et al. (1977)
Locus ceruleus	Total neuron number	24	14 to 87	43.8	48.0	Brody (1978)
Locus ceruleus	Number of neurons/ 20 micron section	25	32 to 93	35.8	47.7	Tomlinson et al. (1981)

Locus ceruleus	Total neuron number	Not stated	Newborn to 80	50.0	50.0	McGeer et al. (1984b)
Abducens nucleus	Total neuron number	20	Newborn to 87	0.0	0.0	Vijayashankar and Brody (1977)
Facial nerve nucleus	Total neuron number	15	22 to 86	18.5	20.0	Maleci (1934)
Facial nerve nucleus	Total neuron number	37	Newborn to 75	0.0	0.0	Van Buskirk (1948)
Ventral cochlear nucleus	Total neuron number	23	4 months to 80 years	0.0	0.0	Konigsmark and Murphy (1970)
Inferior olive	Total neuron number	18	23 weeks to 89 years	0.0	0.0	Monagle and Brody (1974)
Inferior olive	Total neuron number	4	Newborn to 56	0.0	0.0	Moatamed (1966)

[a] Extrapolated directly from raw data or from percentage of cell loss reported. Constant rate of cell loss with age is assumed.

[b] Seventy-seven years represent the mean age of elderly group; mean age of young adult group is not stated in article.

[c] Slab thickness = 1,125 microns, but depth of slab varied from region to region.

[d] Calculated from changes in neuron density and cortical volume with age in a given cortical area (see text).

[e] Initial study was on 20 subjects from newborn to age 95, but our calculations here are based only on subjects aged 16 to 95 years because of objections raised by Hanley (1974).

[f] Initial data showed an increase in neurons in this region with age, but Haug et al. (1983) reported this as rather representing no decrease with age.

more difficult to assess their relative densities; if A and B were observed separately on different days, this might be virtually impossible. One can easily imagine the additional errors when fibers, vessels, and other structures are added to the pictures.

A number of caveats exist in interpreting the results even of quantitative neuropathologic studies:

Cause of Death. Antemortem states of prolonged hypoxia, hypoglycemia, and similar conditions are more likely to cause a loss of certain types of neurons (for example, hypoxia leading to death of Purkinje cells) than sudden accidental death.

The Interval Between Death and Brain Processing. Most neuropathologic studies do not mention the postmortem interval. It is not known what effect, if any, this may have on neuron number in specific areas of the brain.

Secular Acceleration. Some investigators believe that improvements in hygiene, nutrition, obstetrical procedures, and pre- and postnatal care over the past century have resulted in bigger and "better" brains (Miller and Corsellis 1977). This phenomenon has been called *secular acceleration.* Few researchers take this factor into account (the study of Haug et al. being a noteworthy exception) because it is not clear exactly how to incorporate this vari-

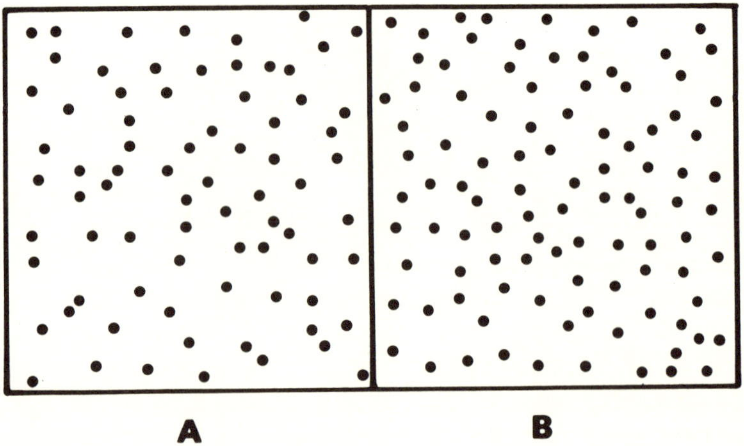

Figure 1. Two different dot densities.

able. On the one hand, the effects of secular acceleration could falsely simulate an aging-related loss of neurons if brains from younger individuals contained more neurons at birth than those of persons born 50 or more years ago. Alternatively, if the major effect of secular acceleration has been an increase in white matter (for example, myelin) rather than grey matter (for example, neurons), then there may be the false appearance of an increase or no change in neuron density with age. Secular acceleration is an important consideration because all neuropathologic studies of human aging have been cross-sectional in nature, longitudinal studies being logistically impractical.

Differences in Gender. Study comparisons must also consider possible differences in the male/female ratio of subjects. Although most studies that have addressed the question of gender differences in age-related neuronal loss have failed to reveal significant differences, this may still be an important factor. For example, there are differences between the mean weights of men's and women's brains at any given age; women's brains generally weigh less. Hence, if women and men have an equal total number of neurons, there would be a greater density of neurons in women than in men. If men and women do not have equal numbers of neurons to begin with, but lose similar numbers over a lifetime, then the percentage loss would be different. Such considerations, although important, have yet to be clarified.

Normality. No brain after death is truly representative of a normal living brain. Only biopsy tissue should be used if measurement of in vivo neuronal populations is desired, but such studies are impractical. Also, postmortem studies draw brains from markedly different populations. Some studies have used brains from institutionalized patients, others have obtained brains through universities or coroners' offices, and these sources are likely to have had different criteria for obtaining and autopsying brains. The medical history of the patients, including a history of alcohol or other drug abuse or the presence of disorders such as mild chronic pulmonary disease, heart failure, or seizures, is often incomplete. The question also arises as to whether many brains from younger age groups are abnormal simply because it is not normal to die at a young age (except perhaps in accidents). Similarly, one may wonder if persons living beyond the age of 90 years are supernormal.

We have touched on just a few of the potentially important variables that are often overlooked in studies of neuron loss with aging. Possible differences relating to race, culture, geographical area, socioeconomic status, and education may also be pertinent. For the present, safety of interpretation lies only with large numbers of studies including large numbers of brains, and the number of both of these has been small. Nevertheless, some tentative inferences may be made based on the studies that have been performed.

NEURONAL LOSS IN NORMAL AGING: A REVIEW

Eight studies have examined the relationship of neuronal loss to aging in the human cerebral cortex (Table 1). Most of these reported an age-related decrease in neuron density of 4 to 6 percent per decade after age 20. Haug et al.'s (1983) study is an exception because they reported an increase in neuron density with age in some areas. However, a concurrent loss of tissue volume in different cortical areas was also found, and in most cases the product of neuron density and volume reveals a decrease in total neuron number with age. In Table 1, cortical areas reported to have an increase in neuronal density with age are designated as showing no change in neuronal number because a true increase in the total number of neurons probably does not occur in the primate central nervous system (Rakic 1985).

Relatively few subcortical structures have been studied (Table 1). We found only one study on the basal ganglia, and this involved only the putamen (Bugiani et al. 1978). Large and small neurons were studied separately, and both appeared to decline in number with age. There has been one study on the amygdala (Herzog and Kemper 1980) that reported phylogenetically older nuclei lost neurons with age, but some of the younger nuclei did not. The hippocampus has been studied, but with conflicting reports. Ball (1977) and Dam (1979) reported a decline in neuron density with age, but Devaney and Johnson (1984) did not find an aging-related loss of nerve cells. We discuss some of our findings on the hippocampus later. Studies of the nucleus basalis of Meynert are difficult to compare. Rogers et al. (1985) and Whitehouse et al. (1983b), whose studies were performed strictly on the nucleus basalis, reported no cell loss with age, but McGeer et al. (1984a) found cell loss in basal forebrain cholinergic cells with age.

The cerebellar cortex, being rather uniform in structure, lends itself well to quantitative studies of Purkinje cell loss with age (Table 1). All studies but one (Delorenzi 1931) reported a Purkinje cell loss with age ranging from approximately a 2.5 percent to 6 percent reduction in neurons per decade. A study on the dentate nucleus (Hopker 1951) failed to show any neuronal loss with age. Our recent studies on changes in Purkinje cell and dentate multipolar cell density with age are discussed later.

Few brainstem nuclei have been investigated quantitatively (Table 1). Brainstem nuclei, being small and relatively discrete, offer advantages for quantitation because the total neuronal population can be estimated with greater accuracy than in larger regions of the brain (see Moatamed 1966). Interestingly, very few studies of brainstem nuclei have demonstrated a loss of neurons with age. Two notable exceptions have been the locus ceruleus and the substantia nigra (Brody 1978; McGeer et al. 1977, 1984b; Tomlinson et al. 1981), two pigmented nuclei that are rich in catecholaminergic neurons. Several studies by Brody (1978) and coworkers (Monagle and Brody 1974; Vijayashankar and Brody 1977) illustrate the difference between a brainstem area rich in catecholamines (locus ceruleus) and two brainstem areas that are not (inferior olive and abducens nucleus). The possible involvement of catecholamines in age-related neuronal loss is discussed later.

QUANTITATIVE NEURONOMETRIC STUDIES OF CEREBELLUM AND HIPPOCAMPUS IN NORMAL HUMAN AGING

Over the past two years, we have been engaged in quantitative studies of age-related changes in neuronal number in the human brain. We initially chose the cerebellum and hippocampus for study, postulating that age-related changes in coordination and memory, respectively, may reflect cell loss in these structures. In this section, we outline the materials and methods we used and briefly review some of our results (see Jeste et al. in press).

Materials

We studied human brains from the "normative" series in the Yakovlev collection at the Armed Forces Institute of Pathology, Washington, D.C. The Yakovlev collection is well known for its high standard of uniformity of processing whole brains. Sections of cerebellum and hippocampus were chosen on the basis of predetermined atlas criteria.

Methods

Blind measurements were taken regarding each subject's clinical autopsy data. Cell counts were done using a Zeiss Videoplan II system, consisting of an electronic planimeter attached to a microcomputer, a light microscope, a television camera, and a video screen. A section under the microscope was magnified and projected onto the video screen, which was connected to a magnetic tablet and the computer. With this technique, each neuron was counted once. Quantitative measurements of the number of neurons per unit area and unit perimeter were obtained. Reliability of cell counts was evaluated by having three investigators independently measure Purkinje cell density in selected sections from the same subjects ($n = 19$). The intraclass correlation coefficient for the values obtained by the three raters was 0.82 ($p < .0001$). Measurements of the density of multipolar cells in the dentate and pyramidal cells in the hippocampus also had highly significant interrater reliability ($p < .0001$).

In the cerebellum, we measured Purkinje cell density (in cells/mm) in the anterior vermis, posterior vermis, and cerebellar hemispheres along with multipolar cell density (in cells/mm^2) in the dentate nucleus. Only those Purkinje cells that displayed a distinct nucleolus were counted. A photomicrograph of a typical folium from the cerebellar hemisphere of a 20-year-old is shown in Figure 2. In the hippocampus, we measured the pyramidal cell density (in cells/mm^2) in regions CA1 through CA4 (these regions are illustrated in Figure 3) (see Mani et al. in press).

For many brains, 40 to 60 sections of cerebellar hemisphere were available. To determine the variability of Purkinje cell density in different sections from the same cerebellar hemisphere, we conducted a pilot study in 12 subjects ranging in age from 10 to 90 years. We examined every second section of cerebellar hemisphere (that is, 20 to 30 sections per subject) and measured Purkinje cell density in several folia in each section. There was a highly significant correlation among the values for neuronal density in folia from different sections of the same subject (intraclass correlation coefficient = 0.79; $p < .0001$).

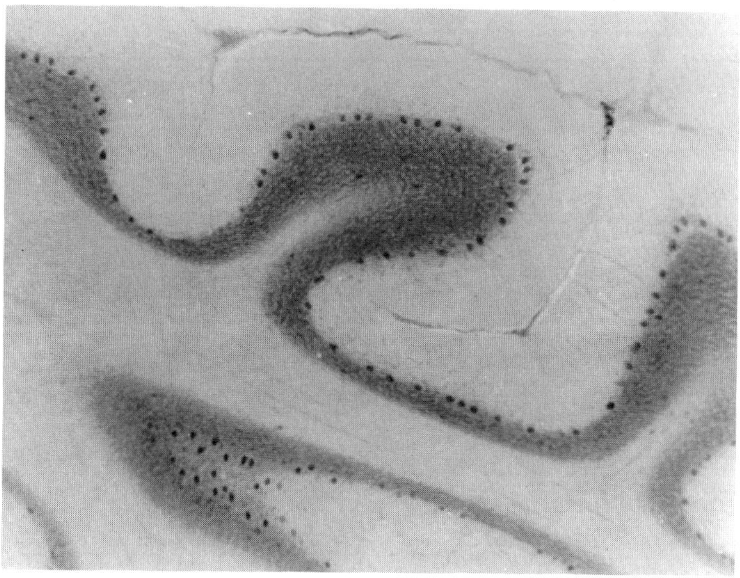

Figure 2. A photomicrograph of a cerebellar folium showing the cerebellar Purkinje cells. The folium is from the cerebellar hemisphere of a 20-year-old man. The Purkinje cell linear density of the central folium is 10.2 cells/mm. Magnification is 40x.

Results

Cerebellum and Aging. We studied 47 normative cerebella from individuals ranging in age from 3 to 98 years. We found a significant negative correlation between age and Purkinje cell linear density in all cerebellar areas investigated, especially in the anterior vermis (Pearson's $r = -.62$, $p < .0001$). No correlation of age with dentate multipolar cell density was found. No differences were found between men ($n = 29$) and women ($n = 18$).

Hippocampus and Aging. We studied right and left normative hippocampi from 23 individuals (age range, 4 to 98 years). No significant correlations with age were found in hippocampal pyramidal cell density nor with pyramidal cell area and nuclear area in regions CA1 through CA3. CA4 cell density showed a significant inverse correlation with age ($r = -.57$; $p < .01$). There were no significant differences between men ($n = 13$) and women ($n = 10$). Subjects over age 65 years ($n = 8$) in general had a lower mean pyramidal cell density than those under 65 ($n = 15$), but this reached significance only in area CA4. This difference was observed on both sides of the brain (left hippocampus:

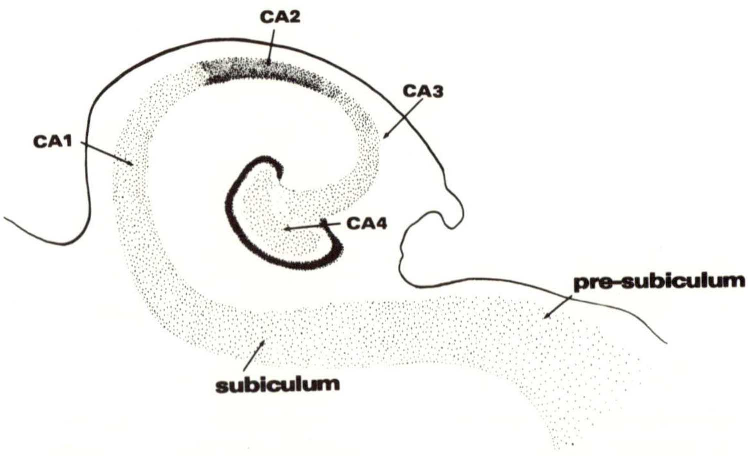

Figure 3. A semischematic diagram of a coronal section through hippocampus showing the different hippocampal fields.

191 ± 36 versus 255 ± 54 cells/mm², $p < .01$; right hippocampus: 188 ± 28 versus 270 ± 70 cells/mm², $p < .005$).

Summary

We found a probable loss of Purkinje cells with age as reflected by a decrease in Purkinje cell linear density with age. In contrast, we could not demonstrate any significant changes in the density of dentate multipolar cells with age. In area CA4 of the right and left hippocampi, subjects over age 65 years had reduced neuronal density when compared with subjects under 65 years of age.

PATHOPHYSIOLOGY OF NEURONAL LOSS WITH AGING: A HYPOTHESIS

A number of hypotheses have been proffered to explain the selective vulnerability of specific brain regions to the effects of aging, including differences in vascular supply, metabolic rate, ontogeny and phylogeny, susceptibility to certain noxious agents (Finch 1976, 1978; Katzman and Terry 1983). None of these hypotheses fully explain the observed variations in aging-associated neuronal loss. We believe that another possible mechanism—selective vulnerability of regions rich in catecholamines—may be important.

Parkinson's disease has long been thought to represent a process of accelerated or exaggerated aging in selected brain areas (Hornykiewicz 1983), stimulating interest in the connection between dopamine and aging. It is now widely accepted that dopaminergic ascending neurons along with postsynaptic dopamine receptors degenerate with age in normal individuals (Hornykiewicz 1983; Memo et al. 1980; Missale et al. 1983; Roth 1983; Severson and Finch 1980). Furthermore, this neuronal loss is accompanied by a decline in dopamine content in the striatum, which may amount to 50 percent by age 65 (Carlsson and Winblad 1976).

The loss of catecholaminergic neurons in humans does not appear to be a simple reflection of generalized neuronal death with age, for, as was pointed out earlier in this chapter, the only brainstem areas that have been consistently shown to have age-related neuronal loss are the substantia nigra and the locus ceruleus, both of which are rich in catecholamines.

The fact that both dopamine neurons and dopamine receptors are lost in normal aging is of interest. Parkinson's disease is associated with a loss of dopaminergic neurons accompanied, at least initially, by a compensatory increase in postsynaptic dopamine receptors. This phenomenon does not occur in normal aging, and both neurons and receptors appear to be lost together. This fact has prompted investigators to consider the possibility that the dopamine neuron terminals may exert a trophic influence on postsynaptic dopamine receptors (Agnati and Fuxe 1980, 1984; Fuxe et al. 1981). It has been shown that levodopa (L-Dopa) administered to mice not only prolongs the longevity of certain strains with very short life spans by as much as 50 percent, but it also enhances their fertility and prevents age-related decreases in motor activity (Cotzias et al. 1977; Papavasiliou et al. 1981), suggesting an antiaging effect of dopamine.

The possibility that dopamine neurons exert a trophic influence in the brain, and that exogenously administered dopamine may increase the life span and preserve function in some strains of mice, prompted us to review the relationship between neuron loss and dopamine content in different areas of the brain. Our hypothesis was that in brain areas richly innervated by dopaminergic neurons the age-related loss of dopamine-containing cells might cause neuronal death by virtue of a loss of trophic influences.

We correlated the neuron loss reported by different investigators for different cerebral cortical areas in humans (discussed earlier in this chapter) with the dopamine content of similar cortical areas in rhesus monkey brains as reported by Björklund et al. (1978). These findings are plotted in Figure 4. There is a significant correlation (Spearman's $r = .62$, $p < .01$) between the percentage of neurons reportedly lost over a 50-year period in humans and the dopamine content in the same areas (although the dopamine measurements had been made in rhesus monkey brains).

Several caveats must be kept in mind regarding this correlation. First, some of the data are from humans and some are from monkeys. Second, the cell loss data are taken from many different studies with differences in methodology. It should be noted, however, that a recent study that examined age-related tissue volume loss in different areas of the human brain reported that the largest losses occurred in the basal ganglia (especially the corpus striatum) as well as in the frontal lobes; there was comparatively little change in volume noted elsewhere. This reported tissue loss coincides with areas of highest dopaminergic input (Haug et al. 1983). Third, neuronal loss has been calculated assuming that neurons are lost at a constant rate throughout life, whereas there is evidence to suggest that, at least in some areas, neuronal loss may occur at a faster rate after the sixth decade (see, for example, the studies of Halle et al. 1975 and Brody 1978). Nevertheless, in most

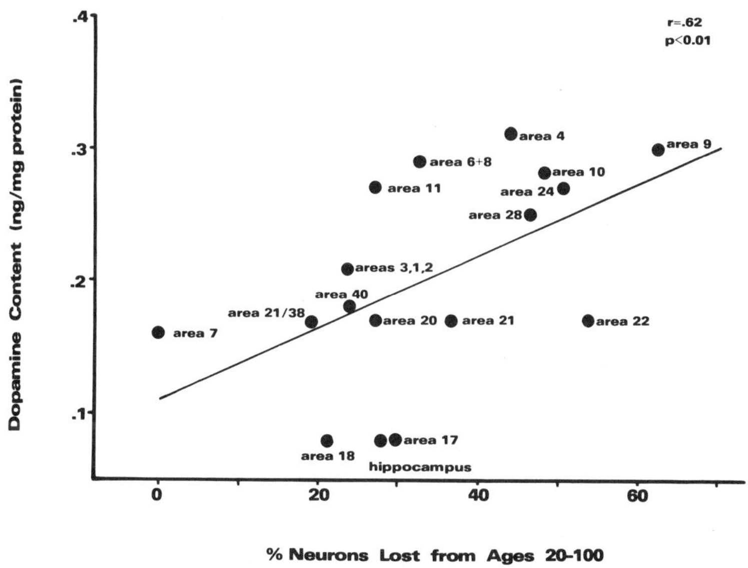

Figure 4. A plot of neuronal loss in human cerebral cortical areas against dopamine content of corresponding areas in rhesus monkey brain. The data for neuronal loss are taken from the studies presented in Table 1 (if more than one set of published data values exist for a given area, the average neuronal loss for the different studies is used in this graph). The data for dopamine content are taken from the study of Bjorklund et al. (1978).

of the studies of cortex reported previously, there is little evidence for assuming that the cell loss is not linear.

If there is a relationship between dopamine and neuron loss, dopamine-mediated trophism is not the only explanation. Rather than exerting a trophic effect, dopamine, or a product of its metabolism, may be toxic to cells. Free radicals have been proposed to be mediators of tissue injury in aging (Cutler 1984; Floyd et al. 1984; Harman 1984; Sohal 1984). Free radicals (of which molecular oxygen, hydroxyl radicals, and superoxide are examples) are chemical compounds that have an odd number of electrons. They are unstable, very reactive, and often difficult to isolate during chemical reactions. They also constitute intermediate species in several biochemical processes. It has been proposed that cytotoxic free radicals generated during the metabolism of dopamine might account for the loss of cells in the substantia nigra in Parkinson's disease, because free radical scavengers (such as glutathione) have been found to be reduced in these patients (Perry et al. 1982). However, in one study, rats given high doses of L-Dopa and carbidopa did not appear to suffer nigral neuron loss (Perry et al. 1984). In this latter study, the attempt to inhibit glutathione was unsuccessful, so it is possible that glutathione and other free radical scavengers were sufficient to prevent neuron damage from free radicals generated from the excess dopamine. The formation of free radicals in dopamine-containing areas may damage neurons over the course of many years, and rats given high doses of L-Dopa over 120 days may not be an appropriate model. These considerations may apply equally well to other catecholamines such as norepinephrine, although previous studies have concentrated mainly on dopamine-related processes.

These hypotheses are consistent with the results of our own studies that were reported earlier in this chapter. For example, it has been demonstrated that there is a direct catecholaminergic input from the locus ceruleus to the Purkinje cells of the cerebellum (see Schulman 1983). The cerebellum also appears to contain lower concentrations of the powerful antioxidant alpha-tocopherol (vitamin E) than other areas of the brain (Halliwell and Gutteridge 1985). In the hippocampus, it has been reported that the largest catecholaminergic input is into the hilus or area CA4 (see Walaas 1983), which is where we observed the greatest decrease in cell density in elderly persons.

Much more research is required to substantiate these hypotheses, but we believe the possibility of a connection between catecholamines and neuron loss, whether the result of trophic or toxic properties of catecholamines, is worthy of further investigation.

NEURONAL LOSS IN DEMENTING DISORDERS

It has been known for many years that certain dementing disorders are associated with gross atrophy and neuronal loss in specific areas of the brain. For instance, Alzheimer's disease is associated with atrophy of cerebral cortex, Parkinson's disease with degenerative changes in the substantia nigra pars compacta, and Huntington's disease with atrophy of the striatum (see the excellent reviews on these subjects by Teravainen and Calne 1983; Terry and Katzman 1983; Wexler 1984). In this section we focus primarily on the loss of cholinergic neurons in the nucleus basalis of Meynert (nbM) in various dementing disorders. Cholinergic mechanisms are considered important in memory and related cognitive functions, although it is likely that noradrenergic and other mechanisms also contribute. The nbM, located in the substantia innominata, is a major source of cholinergic innervation of the cerebral cortex. The cholinergic neurons in the nbM are characterized by their large size, plentiful Nissl substance, and acetylcholinesterase (AChE, the enzyme that metabolizes acetylcholine) activity. As discussed earlier (also, see Table 1), there is some uncertainty about a loss of nbM neurons with normal aging. Recently, Whitehouse et al. (1982) demonstrated a profound (greater than 75 percent) and relatively selective degeneration of cholinergic neurons in the nbM in 5 patients with Alzheimer's disease. This finding provides a pathologic substrate for the marked reduction in the presynaptic markers for cholinergic neurons in the cortex of Alzheimer's disease patients. The loss of nbM neurons in Alzheimer's disease patients has been confirmed by a number of other investigators (for example, Arendt et al. 1983;

McGeer et al. 1984a; Rogers et al. 1985). McGeer et al. (1984a) reported that all the giant cholinergic neurons in the medial basal forebrain (which includes the nbM) decreased from over 400,000 in young controls to about 140,000 in elderly controls. Five patients with Alzheimer's disease had counts between 45,000 and 100,000 neurons. There was a parallel reduction in choline acetyltransferase (ChAT, the enzyme that catalyzes synthesis of acetylcholine) activity in the frontal cortex. The investigators proposed that when the cholinergic cell number in the basal forebrain drops below 100,000 neurons, the cortical ChAT activity may be so low that clinical dementia appears. The relationship of the loss of nbM neurons to a reduction in neocortical ChAT activity was further confirmed when Clark et al. (1983) demonstrated that Huntington's disease was not associated either with a loss of nbM neurons or with a decrease in cortical ChAT activity. Arendt et al. (1983) also failed to find a significant reduction in the nbM cell count in Huntington's disease.

Whitehouse et al. (1983a) reported a selective and significant loss of nbM neurons in 12 Parkinson's disease patients with dementia. The authors proposed that this finding provided an important link between the dementias of Alzheimer's and Parkinson's diseases. The loss of nbM neurons in idiopathic Parkinson's disease has been confirmed by Arendt et al. (1983) (although these researchers found no similar reduction in postencephalitic parkinsonism) and by Rogers et al. (1985). Nakano and Hirano (1983) also found extensive loss of cholinergic neurons in the nbM in two cases of parkinsonism-dementia complex of Guam.

In another study, Nakano and Hirano (1984) questioned the association between depletion of nbM neurons and Alzheimer's disease. These investigators reported that, although there was a significant reduction in the number of nbM neurons in 11 patients with Parkinson's disease, the neuron loss was not associated with other neuropathologic features (such as senile plaques and neurofibrillary tangles in the neocortex, Ammon's horn area, or the nbM) of Alzheimer's disease.

A number of other neuropsychiatric disorders have also been studied from the viewpoint of examining the nbM neuron depletion. Arendt et al. (1983) noted a moderate drop in the number of nbM cholinergic cells in Korsakoff's disease, but no change in schizophrenia, chronic alcoholism without dementia, and infantile brain damage. Rogers et al. (1985) reported a moderate loss of nbM neurons in Creutzfeldt-Jakob disease and in progressive supranuclear palsy, whereas usually nondementing disorders such as multiple sclerosis and amyotrophic lateral sclerosis were not associated with such a depletion.

Thus, it seems that a loss of the large cholinergic neurons in the basal forebrain, especially the nbM, is a feature common to Alzheimer's disease and certain other dementing disorders. It should also be stressed, however, that dementias can occur without a reduction of nbM neurons (for example, Huntington's disease), and conversely a loss of nbM neurons may be present without other evidence of dementia (as in some cases of Parkinson's disease).

Loss of neurons in certain other regions of the brain too may be important in the pathogenesis of dementias. Alzheimer's disease is associated with a significant drop-out of noradrenergic neurons in the locus ceruleus (Bondareff et al. 1982; Iversen et al. 1983), as well as serotonergic neurons in the nucleus raphe dorsalis of the midbrain (Yamamoto and Hirano 1985). Similarly, hippocampal neuronal loss is believed by some investigators to be important in Alzheimer's disease (Ball et al. 1985) and in schizophrenia (Bogerts et al. 1985). Much more work is needed to clarify the contribution of neuronal depletion in selective regions of the brain to specific dementing disorders. With advances in our knowledge in this field, we can hope that, in the near future, it will be possible to arrest, reverse, and even prevent such neuronal loss.

SUMMARY

We have reviewed the literature on neuronal loss in different areas of the brain associated with normal aging as well as certain neuropsychiatric dementias. The field of quantitative neuronometry is young but promising. Several caveats need to be borne in mind when interpreting neuronometric studies. The published literature suggests that the neuronal loss with aging is not uniform but varies greatly in different brain regions. Our own studies of changes in the density of cerebellar Purkinje cells and hippocampal pyramidal cells with aging show considerable interregional differences. We believe that areas with high catecholaminergic innervation may be at a higher risk of neuronal loss in old age. We have discussed possible mechanisms for this selective vulnerability of catecholamine-rich regions to aging-related neuronal dropout. We also have reviewed the evidence for loss of neurons in the nbM in a variety of dementing disorders.

REFERENCES

Agnati LF, Fuxe K: On the mechanism of the antiparkinsonian action of l-dopa and bromocriptine: a theoretical and experimental analysis of dopamine receptor sub- and supersensitivity. J Neural Transm (Supp) 16:69–81, 1980

Agnati LF, Fuxe K: Computer-assisted morphometry and microdensitometry of transmitter identified neurons with special reference to the mesostriatal dopamine pathway. Acta Physiol Scand (Supplement 532): 1–66, 1984

Arendt T, Bigl V, Arendt A, et al: Loss of neurons in the nucleus basalis of Meynert in Alzheimer's disease, paralysis agitans and Korsakoff's disease. Acta Neuropathol 61:101–108, 1983

Ball MJ: Neuronal loss, neurofibrillary tangles and granulovacuolar degeneration in the hippocampus with ageing and dementia. Acta Neuropath 37:111–118, 1977

Ball MJ, Hachinski V, Fox A, et al: A new definition of Alzheimer's disease: a hippocampal dementia. Lancet 1:14–16, 1985

Bayer SA, Hackel JW, Puri PS: Neurons in the rat dentate gyrus granular layer substantially increase during juvenile and adult life. Science 216:890–892, 1982

Björklund A, Divac I, Lindvall O: Regional distribution of catecholamines in monkey cerebral cortex; evidence for a dopaminergic innervation of the primate prefrontal cortex. Neurosci Lett 7:115–119, 1978

Blackwood W, Corsellis JAN: Greenfield's Neuropathology (Third Edition). London, Edward Arnold, 1976

Bogerts B, Meertz E, Schonfeldt-Bausch R: Basal ganglia and limbic system pathology in schizophrenia. Arch Gen Psychiatry 42:784–791, 1985

Bondareff W, Mountjoy CQ, Roth M: Loss of neurons of origin of the adrenergic projection to the cerebral cortex (nucleus locus ceruleus) in senile dementia. Neurology 32:164–168, 1982

Brody H: Organization of cerebral cortex: III. a study of aging in the human cerebral cortex. J Comp Neurol 102:511–556, 1955

Brody H: Structural changes in the aging nervous system, in Interdisciplinary Topics in Gerontology (vol. 7). Edited by Blumenthal HT. New York, Karger, 1970

Brody H: Cell counts in cerebral cortex and brainstem, in Alzheimer's Disease, Senile Dementia and Related Disorders. Edited by Katzman R, Terry RD, Bick KL. New York, Raven Press, 1978

Bugiani O, Salvarani S, Perdelli F, et al: Nerve cell loss with aging in the putamen. Eur Neurol 17:286–291, 1978

Burns BD: The Mammalian Cerebral Cortex. London, Edward Arnold, 1958

Carlsson A, Winblad B: Influence of age and time interval between death and autopsy in dopamine and 3-methoxytyramine levels in human basal ganglia. J Neural Transm 38:271–276, 1976

Clark AW, Parhad IM, Folstein SE, et al: The nucleus basalis in Huntington's disease. Neurology 33:1262–1267, 1983

Colon EJ: The elderly brain. A quantitative analysis in the cerebral cortex of two cases. Psychiat Neurol Neurochir (Amst) 75:261–270, 1971

Comfort A: Neuromythology? Nature 229:282, 1971

Cotzias GC, Miller ST, Tang LC, et al: Levodopa, fertility, and longevity. Science 196:549–551, 1977

Cutler RG: Antioxidants and longevity, in Free Radicals in Molecular Biology, Aging, and Disease: Aging [Volume 27]. Edited by Armstrong D, Sohal RS, Cutler RG, et al. New York, Raven Press, 1984

Dam AM: The density of neurons in the human hippocampus. J Neuropath Appl Neurobiol 5:249–264, 1979

Delorenzi E: Constanza numerica delle cellule di Purkinje del cervelletto dell'uomo, in individui di varia eta. Zeitsch Zellforsch Mikro Anatomie 14:310–316, 1931

Devaney KO, Johnson HA: Neuron loss in the aging visual cortex of man. J Gerontol 35:836–841, 1980

Devaney KO, Johnson HA: Changes in cell density within the human hippocampal formation as a function of age. Gerontology 30:100–108, 1984

Ellis RS: A preliminary quantitative study of Purkinje cells in normal, subnormal, and senescent human cerebella. J Comp Neurol 30:229–252, 1919

Ellis RS: Norms for some structural changes in the human cerebellum from birth to old age. J Comp Neurol 32:1–33, 1920

Finch CE: The regulation of physiological changes during mammalian aging. Q Rev Biol, 51:49–83, 1976

Finch CE: The brain and aging, in The Biology of Aging. Edited by Behnke JA, Finch CE, Moment GB. New York, Plenum Press, 1978

Floyd RA, Zaleska MM, Harmon HJ: Possible involvement of iron and oxygen free radicals in aspects of aging in brain, in Free Radicals in Molecular Biology, Aging, and Disease: Aging (vol. 27). Edited by Armstrong D, Sohal RS, Cutler RG, et al. New York, Raven Press, 1984

Fuxe K, Agnati LF, Kohler C, et al: Characterization of normal and supersensitive dopamine receptors: effects of ergot drugs and neuropeptides. J Neural Transm 51:3–37, 1981

Hall TC, Miller AKH, Corsellis JAN: Variations in the human Purkinje cell population according to age and sex. Neuropath Appl Neurobiol 1:267–292, 1975

Halliwell B, Gutteridge JMC. Oxygen radicals and the nervous system. Trends in Neurosci 8:22–26, 1985

Hanley T. "Neuronal fall-out" in aging brain: a review of the quantitative data. Age and Ageing 3:133–151, 1974

Harman D: Free radicals and the origination, evolution, and present status of the free radical theory of aging, in Free Radicals in Molecular Biology, Aging, and Disease: Aging [Volume 27]. Edited by Armstrong D, Sohal RS, Cutler RG, et al. New York, Raven Press, 1984

Haug H, Barmwater U, Eggers R, et al: Anatomical changes in aging brain: morphometric analysis of the human prosencephalon, in Brain Aging, Neuropathology and Neuropharmacology: Aging [Volume 21]. Edited by Cervos-Navarro J, Sarkander HI. New York, Raven Press, 1983

Henderson G, Tomlinson BE, Gibson PH: Cell counts in human cerebral cortex in normal adults throughout life using an image analysing computer. J Neurol Sci 46:113–136, 1980

Herzog AG, Kemper TL: Amygdaloid changes in aging and dementia. Arch Neurol 37:625–629, 1980

Hodge CF: Changes in ganglion cells from birth to senile death. Observations on man and honeybee. J Physiol 17:129–134, 1894

Hopker W: Das Altern des Nucleus Dentatus. Z Alternforsch 5:256–277, 1951

Hornykiewicz O: Dopamine changes in the aging human brain: functional considerations, in Aging Brain and Ergot Alkaloids: Aging [Volume 23]. Edited by Agnoli A, Crepaldi G, Spano PF, et al. New York, Raven Press, 1983

Iversen LL, Rossor MN, Reynolds, et al: Loss of pigmented dopamine-beta-hydroxylase positive cells from locus coeruleus in senile dementia of Alzheimer's type. Neurosci Lett 39:95–100, 1983

Jeste DV, Barban L, Parisi J. Reduced Purkinje cell density in Huntington's disease. Exp Neurol 85:78–86, 1984

Jeste DV, Lohr JB, Mani R. Quantitative neuropathology and aging, in Proceedings of the 4th World Congress of Biological Psychiatry. New York, Elsevier (in press)

Kandel ER: Brain and behavior, in Principles of Neural Science. Edited by Kandel ER, Schwartz JH. New York, Elsevier, 1981

Katzman R, Terry R: Normal aging of the nervous system, in The Neurology of Aging. Edited by Katzman R, Terry R. Philadelphia, Davis, 1983

Kemper T: Neuroanatomical and neuropathological changes in normal aging and in dementia, in Clinical Neurology of Aging. Edited by Albert ML. New York, Oxford, 1984

Konigsmark BW, Murphy EA. Neuronal populations in the human brain. Nature 299:1335, 1970

Konigsmark BW, Murphy EA: Volume of ventral cochlear nucleus in man: its relationship to neuronal population and age. J Neuropathol Exp Neurol 31:304–316, 1971

Leboucq G: Le rapport entre lipoids et la surface de l'hémisphère cérébrale chez l'homme et les singes. Mem Acad R Med Belg 10:55, 1929

Maleci O: Contributo all conoscenza delle variazioni quantitative delle cellule nervose nelle senescenza. Arch Ital Anat Istolog Patolog 33:883–901, 1934

Mani RB, Lohr JB, Jeste DV: Hippocampal pyramidal cells and aging in the human: a quantitative study of neuronal loss in sectors CA1–CA4. Exp Neurology (in press)

McGeer PL, McGeer EG, Suzuki JS: Aging and extrapyramidal function. Arch Neurol 34:33–35, 1977

McGeer PL, McGeer EG, Suzuki J, et al: Aging, Alzheimer's disease, and the cholinergic system of the basal forebrain. Neurology 34:741–745, 1984a

McGeer PL, McGeer EG, Suzuki J, et al: Cholinergic and noradrenergic systems in aging, Alzheimer's disease and Down's syndrome. Abstracts of the Society for Neuroscience, p 995, 1984b

Memo M, Lucchi L, Spano PF, et al: Aging process affects a single class of dopamine receptors. Brain Res 202:488–492, 1980

Miller AKH, Corsellis JAN: Evidence for a secular increase in human brain weight during the past century. Ann Hum Biol 4:253–257, 1977

Missale C, Govoni S, Castelleti L, et al: Brain neurotransmitter changes in the brains of aged rats, in Aging Brain and Ergot Alkaloids: Aging [Volume 23]. Edited by Agnoli A, Crepaldi G, Spano PF, et al. New York, Raven Press, 1983

Moatamed F: Cell frequencies in the human inferior olivary complex. J Comp Neurol 128:109–116, 1966

Monagle RD, Brody H: The effects of age upon the main nucleus of the inferior olive in the human. J Comp Neurol 155:61–66, 1974

Nakano I, Hirano A: Neuron loss in the nucleus basalis of Meynert in parkinsonism-dementia complex of Guam. Ann Neurol 13:87–91, 1983

Nakano I, Hirano A: Parkinson's disease: neuron loss in the nucleus basalis without concomitant Alzheimer's disease. Ann Neurol 15:415–418, 1984

Papavasiliou PS, Miller ST, Thal LJ, et al: Age-related motor and catecholamine alterations in mice on levodopa supplemented diet. Life Sci 28:1945–1952, 1981

Perry TL, Godin DV, Hansen S: Parkinson's disease: a disorder due to nigral glutathione deficiency? Neurosci Lett 33:305–310, 1982

Perry TL, Yong VW, Ito M, et al: Nigrostriatal dopaminergic neurons remain undamaged in rats given high doses of L-DOPA and carbidopa chronically. J Neurochem 43:990–993, 1984

Rakic P: Limits of neurogenesis in primates. Science 227:1054–1056, 1985

Rogers JD, Brogan D, Mirra SS: The nucleus basalis of Meynert in neurological disease: a quantitative morphological study. Ann Neurol 17:163–170, 1985

Roth GS: Brain dopaminergic and opiate receptors and responsiveness during aging, in Aging Brain and Ergot Alkaloids: Aging [Volume 23]. Edited by Agnoli A, Crepaldi G, Spano PF, et al. New York, Raven Press, 1983

Schulman JA: Chemical neuroanatomy of the cerebellar cortex, in Chemical Neuroanatomy. Edited by Emson PC. New York, Raven Press, 1983

Severson JA, Finch CE: Age changes in human basal ganglion dopamine receptors. Fed Proc 39:508, 1980

Shefer VF: Absolute number of neurons and thickness of cerebral cortex during aging, senile and vascular dementia and Pick's and Alzheimer's disease. Neurosci Behav Physiol 6:319–324, 1972

Shefer VF: Hippocampal pathology as a possible factor in the pathogenesis of senile dementias. Neurosci Behav Physiol 8:236–239, 1977

Sohal RS: Metabolic rate, free radicals, and aging, in Free Radicals in Molecular Biology, Aging, and Disease: Aging [Volume 27]. Edited by Armstrong D, Sohal RS, Cutler RG, et al. New York, Raven Press, 1984

Teravainen H, Calne DB: Motor system in normal aging and Parkinson's disease, in The Neurology of Aging. Edited by Katzman R, Terry R. Philadelphia, Davis, 1983

Terry R, Katzman R: Senile dementia of the Alzheimer type: defining a disease, in The Neurology of Aging. Edited by Katzman R, Terry R. Philadelphia, Davis, 1983

Tomlinson BE, Irving D, Blessed G: Cell loss in the locus coeruleus in senile dementia of Alzheimer type. J Neurol Sci 49:419–428, 1981

Van Buskirk C: The seventh nerve complex. J Comp Neurol 82:303–333, 1945

Vijayashankar N, Brody H: A study of aging in the human abducens nucleus. J Comp Neurol 173:433–438, 1977

Walaas I: The hippocampus, in Chemical Neuroanatomy. Edited by Emson PC. New York, Raven Press, 1983

Wexler N: Huntington's disease, in Neuropsychiatric Movement Disorders. Edited by Jeste DV, Wyatt RJ. Washington, DC, American Psychiatric Press, 1984

Whitehouse PJ, Hedreen JC, White CL III, et al: Basal forebrain neurons in the dementia of Parkinson disease. Ann Neurol 13:243–248, 1983a

Whitehouse PJ, Parhad IM, Hedreen JC, et al: Integrity of the nucleus basalis of Meynert in normal aging. Ann Neurol 14:149, 1983b

Whitehouse PJ, Price DL, Struble RG, et al: Alzheimer's disease and senile dementia: loss of neurons in the basal forebrain. Science 215:1237–1239, 1982

Wilkinson A, Davies I: The influence of age and dementia on the neuron population of the mammillary bodies. Age and Ageing 7:151–160, 1978

Yamamoto T, Hirano A: Nucleus raphe dorsalis in Alzheimer's disease: neurofibrillary tangles and loss of large neurons. Ann Neurol 17:573–577, 1985